PRAISE FOR
An Energy Awakening

"Refreshing and inspiring, Jayne's book will help bring you back to yourself, and in love with life all over again."

- **Mike Dooley,** *NY Times* **Bestselling Author of** *Infinite Possibilities*

"You are holding in your hands a gift that will shift your energy and refocus your attention on the most important asset – **YOU!** Jayne, masterfully invites us to take a look in the mirror, stop making excuses and harness your energy to create the future you truly deserve.

This is more than a book. It's a startling alarm clock to everyone that has been lulled to sleep by hyper-busyness as a way of life. I read Jayne instructions on how to harness my energy and maximize my potential like a hungry animal. I am convinced that Jayne is a new fresh voice ready to hug the world with her words of life. Thank you Jayne. We receive your warm embrace as you guide us toward an inner journey of discover and recovery of our brilliant energy."

- **Simon T. Bailey,** *Brillionaire and author of Release Your Brilliance* – www.simontbailey.com

"Jayne Warrilow's **An Energy Awakening** is a magical blueprint for remembering who we really are - and our energy is the gut and soul of this remembrance. This book is simple. Practical. Wise. Read it at your own peril - because you too will experience your energy in fresh and miraculous ways!"

- **Achim Nowak,** *Founder and President of INFLUENS, Author of Power Speaking: The Art of the Exceptional Speaker*

"If you are ready to start showing up for your own life and stop imitating someone else's, you need to talk to Jayne Warrilow. She will change your energy and change your life."

Rick DiBiasio, *Author* www.middleagedcrazy.com

"*An Energy Awakening* is a "must" read for us all - it's packed full of a lot of common sense, easy to read real life experience, with some simple to understand pointers to help you start making a change in your life today."

- **Andy Hogarth,** *Staffline Group plc*

"*An Energy Awakening* is simply stunning and powerful. No matter where you are in your life journey, Jayne will have you experience a new source of awareness that exists within your time and space, help and make you realize how important it is to balance and maintain your energy, everyday… for the rest of our life. Pure soul food for the mind, just open your heart … and let go. There's no better invitation."

- **Andre Gaumond,** *GBG/Global, Montreal Canada*
Founder, EuroWineClub.com, USA

"Such a beautiful piece of writing, I am lapping it up and want to go back and read it slowly and mindfully. Thank you Jayne, for your boldness and courage. You have shared a piece of you in the writing of this book. You inspire me. I think you and I have the same intention of guiding/inspiring others through our own life experiences, and this you have articulated in a beautifully simple and serene way."

- **Rebecca Perkins,** *Best Knickers Always, passionate about midlife*
www.bestknickersalways.com

"Thought provoking and insightful… Jayne's work advances the work in this critical area from the spiritual and esoteric and into the applied world where all of us might benefit in our everyday lives as we continue our individual paths toward enlightenment."

Jeffrey S. Bondy Ph.D., *Thrive Executive Coaching, Pittsburgh PA*

"If you are noticing that what you have tried in the past just isn't reaching your core, and you are looking for a fresh way to dive a little deeper, this book is an absolute must read... and re-read!

Already an extraordinarily gifted coach, Jayne has discovered a way to communicate a wealth of information on how to dig deep, experience, and utilize that precious energy that we are all born with. Energy that will take us to the next level in a fresh, graceful, and timeless way.

There are some books, (*you know, the books that bring you a different awakening each time you read it*), that you just know will become part of your permanent library - this book has already taken its place in mine!!!"

- **Rachel Ringler,** *CEO and owner, PEP Text* www.peptext.com

"Einstein showed us we are all made up of cells of vibrating energy. Left unmolested, that energy allows for a well-maintained and balanced health, both physically and mentally. Over the years, however, our thoughts, and the words and actions of others knock that energy off balance.

As an expert in how our energy affects our lives, Jayne gives an amazingly honest look at her own journey and the journey all of us are on. She offers simple, practical applications to rebalance and maintain that energy. Jayne's amazing book offers a loving invitation to take control so you too can change your energy to change your world!"

- **Kathy Jo Slusher-Haas,** *Market your Coaching Business*

"There are literally hundreds of personal improvement, self development and how to succeed in business books available, and I have probably read the majority of them. Yet none of them have the missing piece that Jayne provides; How are we showing up in our lives?... Brilliant, simply brilliant! We can't keep pushing forward without learning how to heal from the inside out. Jayne's giving us those tools to change our lives once and for all!"

- **Charlyn Shelton,** *Boomerpreneur/Social Media Concierge, CS Enterprises International Inc.*

"Jayne writes with a humble and humorous eloquence that touches my soul and brings a smile to my heart. The pure wisdom and insight in her words communicate not only her scholarly knowledge but more importantly her own authentic experience of the energetic awakening process. She offers deep soulful material in a most tangible manner, making it accessible to those just stepping onto the path of awakening as well as to those who have been traveling for a while.

Jayne's intention to inspire awareness and joy and her profound yet playful invitation to join her in being a work in progress are embodied in every word. The daily exercises and meditations take the teachings beyond words and into personal experience. They brilliantly encourage self-observation and reflection so that genuine transformation can occur. This offering emanates from a soul who is passionately dedicated to her own awakening process in service to the greater good."

- **Sarah Luna** *MTP, Transpersonal Psychologist/Transformational Coach*

"I simply loved it and really enjoyed the pacing, the observations and the reflections. I have been so very aware of the need to make more space; your writing has just prompted me to leave the chaos that is my life currently and take a moment to breathe, center myself and just be present in the moment. I will definitely be buying **An Energy Awakening** for so many of my friends, who are special in my life because we are sharing a journey towards the promise of being better, being more ourselves. Your ideas and reflections will help us every step of the way"

Lesley-Anne Rutter, *Neuro-physiotherapist & Counsellor*

"An empowering read... I have read a lot of inspirational/self help/development/consciousness books and would not have picked one off the shelf right now, but what I appreciated about *An Energy Awakening* was that it had so so much in every paragraph. Densely packed with wisdom's and reflections, it did inspire me and open up possibilities. I am not one for 'now do this' I have learnt over the years that I just don't do it, however as the book flows over and through you some of those just stick and my mind came back to things that were relevant for me right now. I like the day by day approach. An Energy Awakening has maturity and gains much from the weaving in of your personal story."

Sally Blades, *Acupuncturist & Transformational Coach*

"I have known Jayne now for 3 years and she is on many levels, beyond a coach, a counselor, a mentor, a gifted guide, and a blooming spiritual being. She has personally touched my life on many levels and has skillfully guided me with several personal awakening moments of reflection within my very self, on a spiritual, physical, and mental level.

I would recommend her book *An Energy Awakening* to every human being who, through seeking self, has questioned their soul path, their truest purpose, or has burned the torch to seek a higher meaning in life. Jayne has walked, (and I will personally vouch for), and is still walking and waking to the future of her dreams. And she creates it, where ever she roams. So if one lady has it to say, and can say it best, let it be *Jayne Warrilow* as, in my personal knowing, she has crossed the bridge when there wasn't one in sight, and she moves mountains for others to help them to arise from their struggles, and it all starts within Self. For every crack that may form she will smooth the very surface and make whole again. She will be the inspiration for others and their life purpose. I call her my shining star that never burns out..."

Stormy Lake, *Energy Medicine Practitioner, Divine Energy*
www.divineenergyhealinginc.com

An Energy Awakening...a sacred source of familiar companionship... invites you to simply be present, be in touch with what is authentic and real for you as your own intuitive voice awakens and transforms.

A resonant voice, ***Jayne Warrilow's*** life's calling and inner knowing of what transforms the human spirit radiant's in the pages that unfold. Filled with the essence of wisdom and the relevance of being human this book which will surely engage your soul and energy to refresh, renew, rethink, and recharge!

Annette Hurley, Master Certified Coach, Coaches4Change, LLC

When you are ready, a guide will come and what they have to say is just what you need to hear.

As I read this book, my epiphanies were not in learning anything new, they lay in being **reminded** of all that I had forgotten and all that I could reclaim if I just stopped, took a breath and became honestly present in my life. As I read the book I became reacquainted with someone I hadn't met in a while... me.

Nicholas Warrilow

AN ENERGY AWAKENING

How the power of energy can change your life

JAYNE WARRILOW

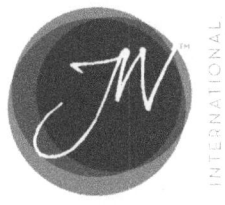

Publisher's Note

This publication is designed to provide accurate and authoritative information in regard to the subject matter covered. It is sold with the understanding that the author is not engaged in rendering psychological, financial, legal or other professional services. If expert assistance or counseling is needed, the services of a competent professional should be sought. The author is not responsible for any errors or omissions, or for the results obtained from the use of this information.

Distributed internationally by the Jayne Warrilow International LLC

Copyright © 2011-2012 by Jayne Warrilow International LLC

ISBN : 978-1-947285-01-9

All rights reserved. No part of this publication may be reproduced, stored in a retrieval system, or transmitted in any form, or by any means, electronic, mechanical, photocopying, recording or otherwise, without the prior written permission of the author (except by a reviewer who may quote brief passages). Printed in the United States of America.
For information and enquiries please contact Jayne Warrilow International LLC.

For more information about the Jayne Warrilow International companies:

      www.JayneWarrilow.com

Library of Congress Cataloging-in-publication Data
Warrilow, Jayne
An Energy Awakening : how the power of energy can change your life / Jayne Warrilow

ISBN : 978-1-947285-01-9

To Mum and Dad...

Who taught me more than they know

With all my love

Contents

Acknowledgements   15
Foreword   17
An Invitation   21

Part One: Finding Self

Day 1: Becoming   29
Day 2: It's okay you can stop now...   31
Day 3: Your calling   33
Day 4: Simplicity   35
Day 5: Developing presence   37
Day 6: Acceptance   39
Day 7: Getting to what matters   41
Day 8: Truth   43
Day 9: Be yourself   45
Day 10: Inner voices   47
Day 11: Space in between   49
Day 12: Fear   51
Day 13: Remembering to breathe   53
Day 14: Trust   55
Day 15: Feeling safe and secure   57
Day 16: Getting out of your head   59
Day 17: Not knowing   61
Day 18: Rest and renewal   63
Day 19: The confidence to create   65
Day 20: Coming home   67

Part Two: Healing the Past

Day 21: Legacies from the past   73
Day 22: Courage   75
Day 23: In the shadow   77
Day 24: Feeling your feelings   79
Day 25: The power of optimism   81
Day 26: Where we've been   83

Day 27: When life is hard   85
Day 28: The night sky   87
Day 29: When you're feeling stuck   89
Day 30: Emptiness   91
Day 31: Frustration   93
Day 32: Cleaning your wounds   95
Day 33: After the pain   97
Day 34: A little more attention   99
Day 35: Letting go   101
Day 36: Wounded heart   103
Day 37: Balanced energy   105
Day 38: Water   107
Day 39: The risk to bloom   109
Day 40: Love   111

Part Three: Finding Freedom

Day 41: Getting real   117
Day 42: Passion   119
Day 43: No need for approval   121
Day 44: The lost art of wanting   123
Day 45: Your infinite energy   125
Day 46: Stop the world   127
Day 47: Moment to moment   129
Day 48: Playing small   131
Day 49: Open your mind   133
Day 50: Knowing   135
Day 51: A blossoming heart   137
Day 52: Leaning into flow   139
Day 53: Forgiveness   141
Day 54: Surprise   143
Day 55: The gift of choice   145
Day 56: Whole body listening   147
Day 57: Stepping into your power   149
Day 58: Unconditional love   151
Day 59: Silence   153
Day 60: Living life out loud   155

Part Four: Beyond The Ego

Day 61: Patience	161
Day 62: Friends	163
Day 63: Mindfulness	165
Day 64: No resistance	167
Day 65: Your vision	169
Day 66: Gratitude	171
Day 67: Your creative DNA	173
Day 68: The art of living	175
Day 69: Healing ourselves	177
Day 70: Your personal vibration	179
Day 71: Your inner leader	181
Day 72: Intuition	183
Day 73: Legacy	185
Day 74: Contribution	187
Day 75: Opening your eyes	189

Part Five: Awakening

Day 76: Inner peace	195
Day 77: Showing up	197
Day 78: Becoming whole	199
Day 79: Honesty and Integrity	201
Day 80: Life as a teacher	203
Day 81: Knowing why	205
Day 82: Living on the edge	207
Day 83: Resonant energy	209
Day 84: Believing	211
Day 85: One-ness	213
Day 86: Earth	215
Day 87: Following the light	217
Day 88: A sense of purpose	219
Day 89: Dare to dream	221
Day 90: A life worth living	223
Epilogue	227
About the Author	229

Recorded by the author, '**An Energetic Journey**'
is a free Guided Meditation that accompanies this book.

For your copy, go to: **https://rebrand.ly/AEA-Meditation**

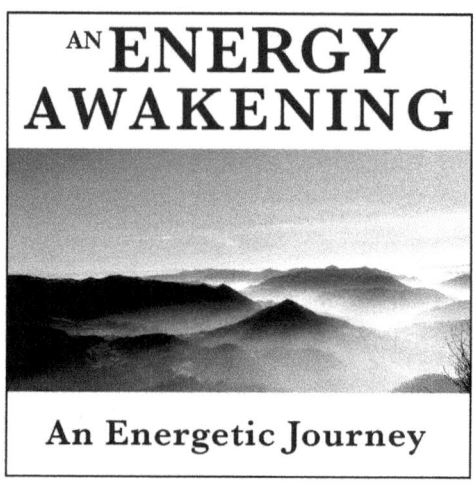

Acknowledgements

First and foremost I want to thank all of my clients and everyone who has ever attended one of my workshops, for their trust, for the honor of being part of their personal journey and for teaching me what works to nurture their energy and their personal and professional growth. It has been my sincere privilege to work with you all, and without your courage and the power of energy awakened within you, this book would not have been possible.

I want to show a deep appreciation to my family who invest their energy with me every day, even when I am totally drained and have nothing left for them. You are my inspiration and the re-energizers within my life:

Nick, you place the solid ground beneath my feet.
Gemma, you embody the energy of love at a level I can only imagine. I will miss your smile more than you know.
Katie, you light up my life showing me anything is possible.
Jakob, you have more energy and zest for life to keep me smiling when the day is long.
To my family back in England who might now understand something more of what it is I do!
To all my clients who kept on asking me to write this book.
To my dog, Milo, whose insistent whining reminded me to take a break and refresh my energy when in the depths of writing...
To Clare for being my best and only sister. I miss you.
To Mark for being the brother I never had.
To Gillian, my bestest friend in the whole wide world.
To Danny for her love and insatiable passion for everything I do.

I want to honor and give thanks to the presence of others who helped me find the space and the energy to shape my thoughts into this book:
Anne Wilson for her belief in me.

Charlyn Shelton for her motivation and encouragement.
Rachel & Gary Ringler - seriously where would I be without you guys?
Stormy Lake for her divine energy and ability to listen from her heart.
Linda Barnby for her friendship and business advice.
Nancy Bevers for her spiritual guidance and soul connection.
Star Ladin for her courage and unwavering support.
Annette Hurley for her vision and passion for energy in life
Achim Nowak for his inspiration.
Andre Gaumond for his advice and encouragement.
Nic Askew for daring me to come out of the closet and step beyond the impersonation.
Susan Harrow for guiding me through my culture shock on first landing in the US and for giving me the texts to inspire me to write.

To all my friends back in England and from all over the world, who have been so patient, so loyal and continue to support me on my journey.
You know who you are...

To all of you who dare to dream of a bigger life... your energy is waiting to show you the way.

Foreword
by Susan Harrow,

author of *Sell Yourself Without Selling Your Soul*

In our ever increasing pace of life never have the words *slow down* been as desperately needed as they are now.

In *An Energy Awakening* Jayne Warrilow takes us by the hand and shows us how to decrease the speed of our lives in order to find our true inner pace.

Indira Gandhi said, "*You must learn to be still in the midst of activity and to be vibrantly alive in response.*" Jayne takes us to this stillness in order that we can find the aliveness ringing through our bodies ourselves, so we can follow the path of most meaning and ultimately nourish and serve others with what makes us come wildly to life.

Often when people talk about energy they are referring to their physical vitality, their Mojo, but Jayne goes deeper than that. She trains us to harness what we have and invest it in living the life we have consciously and carefully set out for ourselves, despite our patterning and programming from our lineage, or pressure from the outside to follow a path not of our own making.

As an executive coach and leader in the global evolution her work in the C-Suites of global organizations is changing the face of leadership as we know it. With her help executives are now beginning to understand the power of their own energy and developing their leadership from the inside out.

Now Jayne is bringing these teachings out from behind the walls of corporations and companies and putting them into the hands of individuals and entrepreneurs so they can learn the secrets to exploring and expressing their deepest inner resources. This fascinating book will act as your guide, no matter who you are or what stage you are currently at in your life. Jayne will show you how to overcome blockages in your energy so you can learn for yourself how to move into balance, alignment and flow.

Enjoy...

CHANGE YOUR ENERGY
AND IT WILL
CHANGE YOUR WORLD

An Invitation

This book is meant to be a companion to you, a soul friend. It is a book about energy awakening. To write this I've had to live it. It has given me the opportunity to go back through many different points in my life, particularly my own healing journey and gather together the many pebbles scattered along my path which have helped, supported, guided and inspired me. It is these that I would like to share with you.

Most of us don't have enough space in our lives to simply be. We are living in times of overwhelming busyness and distraction. We find ourselves caught up in some kind of endless doing. We train ourselves to focus so that we can continue *to do* for extraordinary lengths of time in order for us to *have* more and maybe at some distant point in the future we will eventually find the time to *be*. This seems backwards to me and it is our energy that is suffering. As we find the space in our lives to become quiet enough to listen to the longings of our soul, we arrive at a deeper sense of awareness, one that invites us to appreciate the fullness of who we really are.

I know that a book is only words on a page, but words have energy. Books have the power to take us to many different places, in this dimension and even beyond. I would like you to consider this book as an awakening, a catalyst enabling you to open your eyes just a little wider. It is an introduction to your energy, to exploring the whole of you in ways you may not have previously considered and ultimately I hope it helps you to find your place in the world.

It has been an interesting process for me writing out the explicit entries for you in this book. At certain parts within the writing I became aware that I don't live everything I was writing about. There were times when I was reminded of a long lost insight which had served me so well in the past but had become buried under a mountain of new and more exciting concepts. And when writing about presence, I felt slightly hypocritical because how could I write a piece which clearly advocates the power of presence when much of the time I'm not present myself?

However in the writing, I have been reminded once again that we are all a work in progress and this book offers us all a radical possibility to awaken to our energy, our vitality and harness it to maximum advantage within our lives.

I also caught myself deep within the experience of "flow" a few times, where the outside world seemed to have melted away and the words flowed from somewhere (who knows where?) directly onto the page on my computer screen. And that was sometimes as startling as it was joyful! It reminded me how important it is for me to be able to articulate my passion for energy within my creative expression, and the joy is implicit within the sharing.

My intention with this book is to inspire you to become more aware, more conscious of yourself and your energy. I invite you to come to your learning edge and explore with passion what maybe possible for you. I might even dare to believe that somewhere within you may find your higher calling; a call towards whatever you may have dared or double-dared yourself to do for as long as you can remember. Perhaps now is the time for you to feel compelled to follow.

As you read through these pages, you will find that you know much more than you thought you did on some very deep subjects. The fact is, you already know how to awaken your energy, you have just become distracted and disoriented somewhere along life's path. Once you can reconnect to your energy, you will realize that you have the ability to not only find yourself, but also to free yourself and others. Whether you choose to do so or not is entirely up to you. However as you complete your journey through this book you will know at a deeper level that there is no more hiding, no more confusion, no more blaming others. You will know exactly what you must do.

It is my profound hope that something within the pages of this book will re-energize you, recharge your spirit and help you to live life a little larger, love with more abandon and ultimately find your way to joy.

So it is in the spirit of joy and humility that I invite you to join me in being a work in progress yourself. Take yourself lightly and you will find that the energy flow will find you. Play. Experiment. Have fun. Laugh at yourself along the way. And know that you already know everything you need to awaken your energy and become the strong clear vibration which will fuel not only your personal evolution but the energetic evolution which is building throughout the world.

It is with much love and positive energy, I bring forth my experience of *An Energy Awakening*...

Jayne

*The journey begins right here, in the middle of the road, right beneath your feet.
This is the place.
There is no other place, no other time.*

- N.J. Adler

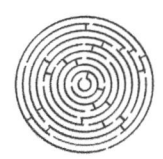

Part One: Finding Self

Adventure is not outside; it is within.

- David Grayson

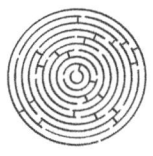

Day 1
Becoming

I am not what happened to me, I am what I chose to become.
- Carl Jung

Why is it so easy for us to live according to what other people want and expect? Why is it so effortless for us to give away our power and live a life someone else wants us to live?

Part of the reason of course, lies in the many pressures we all face in our every day lives. It is too easy to forget ourselves in the hustle and bustle of all the things which need to be done, achieved and ticked off our to-do-list. Who we are today is the clearest indicator of who we are becoming.

There comes a time in all our lives when we begin to wonder about ourselves; the inner person who resides deep within. It is an inescapable quest for *the truth* that lies within us at the heart of our very soul. An essential part of being human. It is an adventure which can lead us down many different paths, uncover countless dimensions of the truth, until one day we rest in the knowledge that what we know about our inner self, for now at least, is enough.

Most of us live our lives *standing outside of ourselves*, ready to judge our physical bodies, our feelings and our thoughts from an external standard. Practically everyone I know and every client I have ever worked with, has lost track of themselves at some point in their life. This is true of myself too. There was a time when I found it easier to listen to the people around me to discover what would be the right decision, or the best way forward for me. I gave more credence to the views of others than finding the space to listen to my own intuitive voice which remained hidden deep inside of me. I defined myself through the feedback from others and lost myself along the way. I accommodated, shaped and molded myself to serve others, often at my own expense. I was too busy in the doing to ever wonder about who I was being.

Let me share a buddhist teaching that asks us to be mindful of how rare it is to find ourselves as a human on Earth. It requests that you look about you and notice the many other forms of life around you, the bird and the butterfly, the loyal dog and the fierce tiger, to the one hundred year old oak and the ancient mountain. It asks us to understand that no other life form has the consciousness of being that we are privilege to.

Just think about it for a moment, of all the many different species of plants, animals and minerals that make up the Earth, it is only us as humans who can enjoy the wakefulness of spirit we know as being conscious. And you and I were both lucky enough to have been born human. You could have been a fly, I could have been a spider. But we were blessed, that in this time and in this place we would be alive in ways we often take for granted.

Be *grateful* for who you are today. Notice how you feel. Go within and reconnect to your inner self, find your inner voice and listen to what it has to say. Explore who you are and who you are becoming.

- *Go for a walk outside and notice all the life which is around you*

- *Breathe slowly and consider all of the other life forms you come across - what can you do that they can't?*

- *Count your blessings.*

- *So what will you do with this day, knowing that you are one of the lucky ones who gets to make a conscious choice?*

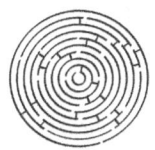

Day 2
It's okay you can stop now...

For fast acting relief, try slowing down. Lily Tomlin

So what happened? When did our lives become so busy? How did we fill our days with so many things? Too much of everything is like a modern sickness, it can be distracting and put us under unnecessary amounts of pressure.

Many of us spend our days racing to catch up with ourselves. There are ever increasing demands being made on our time and it can be difficult to know where to turn and what to do next. As we are pulled in different directions we are also confronted with the ever-growing list of ways to communicate with our nearest and dearest, with iPhones, Blackberries, texts, and emails, not to mention Facebook and other social networking sites. They all seem to accelerate our stress rather than improve the quality of our relationships. Couple this with the ambition many of us have to lead a successful life and we are well on our way to burn-out.

Despite the fact that many of us have way too much going on in our lives, in my role as a coach I still meet people on a daily basis who want more. More freedom, more love, more confidence, more energy, more sales, more money, more time, you name it... someone somewhere will want more of it. The irony is the solution to our need for more often entails doing *less*.

The more we have in our lives the more successful many of us think we'll be, but the exact opposite is often true. In what has been termed the "paradox of choice" a large amount of choices can become overwhelming instead of liberating. If we have too many choices we end up feeling out of control. In order to avoid the panic of being too busy to think we need to give ourselves *permission to stop*. Often when we feel overwhelmed our natural instincts are to tell ourselves to try harder, "pull ourselves together" and carry on regardless. This exacerbates the problem and only makes us feel much worse. This is when we need to take a breath and stop. We need to come back to our core and regain our sense of balance.

When we *slow life down*, it is much easier for us to be in touch with what is authentic and real. It takes a certain amount of courage to truly do nothing, even if only for a short time. We get drawn into the external activity of life and we also become entangled in the inner tangle of our constant thoughts and judgements. It can be an act of courage to simply let go of life and sit still. Rest. Be. Do absolutely nothing. It can be one of the most challenging and rewarding things a human being can do and now it's your turn. Find some space in your life today, and just be.

- *Center yourself by breathing steadily, relax into your breath*
- *Meditate on the pace at which you live your life - how would you benefit from slowing down?*
- *If you take a step back from your life - what do you notice?*
- *Are you living the life you want to live? If not, what one small step can you take today in the right direction?*
- *How can you regain your center of balance?*
- *Be still in the moment. Be.*

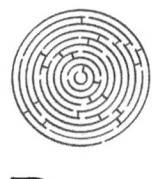

Day 3
Your calling

Changing your life is an inside job.

What feels like a hundred years ago, somewhere in a busy street in the middle of London, a part of the invisible world was made, for just a brief moment, visible to me. I saw the light streaming through the trees, dancing off the car rooftops and the energy rising from the crowd rushing home after a long day's work. I saw great streams of colorful energy everywhere around me, each particle containing essential information radiating out into the Universe. I knew at that moment that life was far greater, far more expansive, far more amazing than my mind could grasp. *Everything was alive with energy* and I was an essential part in this vibrant, energetic world. I was awake for just a brief moment.

Many years later, laying prostrate in a hospital bed I remembered. I realized that my light was dimming, and that my own body was literally flooded with energy of which I was only dimly aware. I remembered that there was energy all around me which I needed to harness for my own well-being. It seemed to tug at my knowing, touching me somewhere deep inside, prompting me to take the necessary steps back to health. It was not going to allow me to continue to sleep my way through this lifetime. It was simply my wake-up call, encouraging me to remember that which I already knew. What will be yours? What is it that you need to remember that you have long forgotten? What will be your call to wake up and be a larger contribution to the world? It may be a call to do something; it may be time for you to move into action, to change your career, forgive your parents or leave a relationship. Or you may be called to be something; more loving, less fearful, more appreciative, less demanding. You may feel called to move towards something or even away from something. You maybe called to retreat, stand back and reflect. You may be called to teach. You maybe called to live your childhood dreams, to dare to take the first step upon the path of living your destiny.

I'm not sure if we do really forget our callings or if we simply fear what might happen if we pursue them. I think we might also fear raising our hopes of envisioning a better future, what if we dare to dream, unleashing our deepest desires only in reality to be left broken and disappointed upon the shores of our own longings? There are a multitude of forces which conspire against us. I know saying "yes" to my calling plunged me into a deep inner conflict where part of me knew it didn't make any sense whatsoever, (I felt called to heal which the doctors told me was impossible) yet another part of me knew my life wouldn't make sense without it.

There are no guarantees. *Your calling doesn't come gift wrapped announcing its arrival in your life with a fanfare of trumpets.* You need to listen and be awake to hear your call. It can come in many disguises. You need to be open to read the signs. Calls are often questions to which you need to respond, reveal your vulnerability to and stand naked before. They shake you loose from your moorings, knock you off your ground to prepare you for important changes which you can't see or even imagine yet. Yet they reignite a spark, lighting a fire deep within in your belly that can be difficult, if not impossible to ignore.

- *Sit quietly, contemplate the possibility that there is a calling waiting for you*
- *Open your mind and reflect upon what that might be*
- *How open do you sense yourself being? How patient?*
- *How might you be failing to notice the signs?*
- *Know that with rhythm and right timing, when you are ready, your calling will find you*

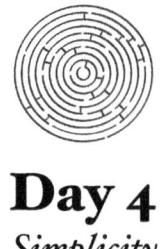

Day 4
Simplicity

We have to live and we have to die; the rest we make up.
- Anon

Whatever happened to leading a simple life? So many of us have trained ourselves to want the best in life that we can overcomplicate things often without realizing it. I remember being in a restaurant with a friend who wouldn't accept her drink unless it was made with a particular brand of vodka. She was in fact, quite indignant about it. Or going to Starbucks with another friend who had to have their coffee served up in a complex and special way, as if this need to be different was an integral part of her identity to be shared publicly wherever she went. Or coaching a very lonely client whose criteria for partnership was so exceptional no-one could possibly meet their expectations. I used to maintain similar high standards until my illness taught me otherwise.

The *devastating truth* is that when you are bed-ridden, being demanding or sophisticated doesn't help you to survive. It only makes you a difficult patient and alienates you further from the glimpses of humanity that you miss from your normal life.

The simplicity of daily life is what I missed. I begin to notice the concerned looks of everyone who visited from my family and friends, to the doctors in charge and I hungered for the simplicity of a normal day. I longed for the feeling of the sun on my face, the wind in my hair and the carefree laughter of friends. I yearned for some semblance of health, for a day free from pain and a night well slept. Things we take for granted on a daily basis became like diamonds just out of reach.

There lies a profound insight in the fact that I, like an innocent child, became easily pleased with whatever simple gifts each day brought. I counted the days back to normal. I knew that each day in pain, was another behind me, one step closer to my recovery. And so began my waking into life.

The further I journey the more I realize that the extraordinary lies in the simplicity of what is ordinary. Our unique demands do not signify a level of importance, they merely mask the insecurities within. I have learned to accept whatever life brings my way knowing that there is as much value in the pain as well as the joy, there is as much light in the broken bottle as there is in a diamond ring. And it is simplicity that clears my vision enabling me to see into the depths of my soul and remember at my very core, what it is that really matters to me.

- *Find some space to relax and breathe deeply. Remember a time when you were particularly demanding*
- *Meditate on what you were truly asking for by being so demanding*
- *If you needed love, release that need now and commit to loving whatever comes into your life*
- *If you needed to be seen as special, breathe out and know deep within that you already are unique and special*
- *If you needed someone's attention, accept that need now and with your next breath, pay attention to whatever is near*
- *As you go through your day take responsibility for radiating out to others whatever you have identified that you need*
- *Know that within time this will be returned to you threefold.*

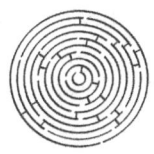

Day 5
Developing presence

Whatever the present moment contains accept
it as though you chose it.
- Eckhart Tolle

Whether you know it or not your already have all the freedom you could ever desire. And you have it right now in this present moment. You are not yet in tomorrow and no longer in yesterday, you are here now and you are free to do with this moment what you want. True freedom comes from how you respond to your life and not what your life does to you. *You choose* how to respond to what your life puts in front of you. *You choose* how to understand it. *You choose* how to feel about it. *You choose* what to do with it. *You choose* whether to react or respond to the challenging situations that confront you. When you learn how to stop habitually reacting and start consciously responding to the events and people in your life you become truly independent, truly powerful and truly free and you live your life from a place of presence.

Presence is magnetic. Others notice you and want to spend more time with you. Have you ever noticed how difficult it is to remain unconscious when you are around someone who is present, aware and connected? Becoming present yourself, acts as an unseen invitation to others around you to step into the present moment with you. It takes them out of their heads and brings them back into their physical bodies, to notice the current situation in the here and now instead of lamenting the past or worrying about the future. By becoming present you raise your energetic frequency and others will respond.

Becoming present not only has benefits for the quality of your life but it also has a profound affect on your others around you. When you are present you are maximally resourceful and responsive to what your circumstances require of you. It is through a commitment to living in the now that you choose, in each living moment, who you are and how you respond to life.

Your inner state is not an accident. When you fully embody who you are in an authentic and genuine manner, you will draw more deeply on your intuition, awareness and energy field to be more effective and more content in your life. Presence is a state of being in which you can live to your full potential. It is a state available to you at any given moment; you only need set the intention and choose.

- *Center yourself, breathe steadily and reflect upon the following:*
- *Remember a time when you had an experience of presence, where you felt moved by a sunset, a waterfall or a spectacular view. What was that feeling like? What did it feel like to be present? How do you know when you are present?*
- *Remember a time when you felt an overwhelming wave of love for someone. What happened in that experience?*
- *Remember a time when you were with someone who was very upset, grief stricken or hurt. A time when your intuition led the way and you understood that you needed to remain calm and hold the space for that person. How did you access that state of calm? How did you hold the space?*
- *Reflect back upon what presence feels like for you. How do you know when you are present and more importantly how do you catch yourself when you're not?*

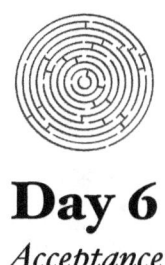

Day 6
Acceptance

It doesn't matter what we do until we accept ourselves.
Once we accept ourselves, it doesn't matter what we do.
- Charly Heavenrich

Accept yourself. If you don't, how can you expect anyone else to? One of the most important relationships you can build in your life is to get to know yourself warts and all. To know your light and your shade, your yin and yang, strengths and weaknesses and to accept everything that you find. You can't go back and change anything, *what is done is done,* so you are left with yourself exactly as you are. Wherever you go in life, there you will be! You don't have to strive or change yourself to achieve perfection, it's actually quite the opposite - you just need to accept yourself in all your wondrous glory.

If there are aspects of you that you want to change, don't beat yourself up over it (we all have them!) *Change what you can and let go of the rest.* Time is short. There is no need to keep berating yourself about what you don't like or to keep living in a way which is out of alignment with your soul. Every dawn is a new day, a new perspective for you to become the best you can be. Another opportunity to embrace a greater level of acceptance of yourself. A day to remember the light within and allow it to shine out.

In reality, there's no way you'll have enough time to live all of your dreams or to reach your full potential, it is simply one of those facts you can't escape. You may not live up to your own high standards, (or someone else's) but you do your best. *Accept this.* You have light and shade within, that is what makes you whole. *Change is inevitable -*

stop resisting and surrender to the flow of your life. The most contented people I have met are those that know this deep within their soul and they pay attention to what they have some control over. They accept themselves and their lives in the present moment and simply let go of the rest. They dedicate themselves to those areas of their life where they can make a difference, where they can change things, where they have some degree of influence and where they will be most fulfilled personally. It is in these places that they live their lives, allowing them to maximize their impact and enjoyment from life.

Don't waste another day without acceptance. Accept yourself now and begin to have the life you aspire to by accepting the life you have.

- *This is a daytime meditation. Sit quietly inside, next to a window if you can and notice the natural light entering your room*
- *Watch the light outside as it moves through trees, through the glass of your window and into your room*
- *Breathe deeply and feel the quality of the light*
- *When the time feels right, keep breathing deeply, walk outside and into the light*
- *Move directly into a patch of sunlight. Inhale deeply and feel its warmth covering your body. Feel it wrap itself around you like a blanket of heat and light.*
- *Stay there.*

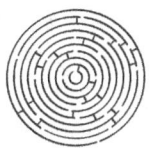

Day 7
Getting to what matters

You come first. Others come second. Results come third.

Meditation is a well recognized technique for energizing, calming and clarifying the mind. It offers you a process to get in touch with your energy and stay connected to whatever matters most to you in the present moment. It's purpose is to learn to focus the attention and to train the mind to enter subtler states of consciousness, transcending the many concerns, worries and anxieties which usually occupy the mind, allowing us to reach deeper and more expansive states of awareness. *It is within meditation that we can begin to unpack our internal landscape and get to what matters.* Of all the methods which are available for developing energetic awareness, meditation is perhaps the most potent. Those who practice meditation regularly report an increased level of functioning in many aspects of their life including better physical health and well-being, less stress, greater productivity in their work, improved concentration, higher levels of creativity and overall more personal satisfaction with their lives. I can speak from personal experience also, as my meditative practice is so important to me, as a mother of three and a busy business owner and coach, my meditation time is *my* time - it simply grounds me and creates space in my hectic (sometimes chaotic) life. It has also been a critical element in my own healing journey and probably one of the most powerful tools for managing my ongoing health condition and its related pain.

Meditation is a journey through the layers of your mind and emotion, sinking beneath into the still, calm, silent place within the very core of your self and your energy. *Storms can rage on the surface of your life, but your core energy is always calm.* The more you shift your focus inwards the more you will discover that the internal self is not just one single destination; you will discover that the edges of who you are, are less rigid than you thought. The deeper you go the more you realize that who you are is actually bigger than you thought and at the very deepest levels the experience of being separate begins to disappear. The ideas of "you" and "me" become blurred, as you begin to experience there is no difference between who you are and who others are, as we are all connected.

There are many techniques for achieving a meditative state, and it is worth trying a few to see which will suit you. Many individuals who are coming to meditation for the first time find it easier to begin by following guided meditations, where you merely need to listen intently and follow instructions. Others may find it easier to just sit with themselves becoming more mindful. And you can do this on your own or within a group setting. Use your intuition and choose the option that appeals to you most. Here are some different techniques to bring you into a meditative state:

- *Regulating and watching one's breath*
- *Focusing on an image e.g. a flame of a candle, a mandala or a symbol*
- *Simply following one's thoughts wherever they may lead*
- *Walking silently and mindfully*
- *Listening intently e.g. to the sounds in your environment, or to a particular music track*
- *Relaxing and allowing yourself to be receptive to whatever comes through*
- *Uttering a mantra or affirmation repeatedly*
- *Running energy by visualizing it moving up and down your body*
- *Observing as a witness*
- *Concentrating on a single concept or problem (e.g. using a Zen koan - what is the sound of one hand clapping?)*
- *Guided visualizations or trance journeys*

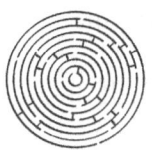

Day 8
Truth

Whoever sets himself up as a judge of truth and knowledge is shipwrecked by the laughter of the Gods.
- Albert Einstein

The truth is your energy matters. When your energy is out of balance so is your life. You can't balance your energy without clear energetic boundaries, in other words you need to be clear about what you will and will not do. Our days can be ruled by random forces. If you spend all your time responding to others' needs and crises, you'll never get time to think about what is really important to you. *Poor energetic boundaries drain your vitality.*

80% of all the problems I encounter with coaching clients are connected to poor energetic boundaries. They are living up to what they think others expect of them, filled with unspoken contracts from their parents, their spouse and other influential people in their lives. They have lost their sense of self along the way. If you are busy living someone else's life who exactly is going to live yours? Let yourself off the hook. Give yourself a break. Allow your inner critic the night off to rediscover your true authentic self. Simply being, rather than being busy, is difficult but it is rewarding. It is however, something you should aspire to every day. How else will you know what is true for you?

Once you build a relationship with your true authentic self you get in tune with your own intuitive energy system. This gateway of information which embraces so many different aspects of who you are from your personality to your values, your behaviors to your beliefs and aims to make more of your unconscious, conscious. You become clear about your energetic boundaries and able to shift into balance. This gives you the potential to keep your head while all around you are losing theirs; to keep yourself on an even keel.

The simplest boundary to put in place is simply learning to say "no". Let's face facts, it can be challenging for most of us to say no; we would rather be nice. This is sad but true. Saying yes and then getting resentful is not good, it affects your energy and can even result in you disturbing your physical energy so much that it results in illness. I have worked with many individuals who struggle to say no to such an extent that their body has begun to say it for them. Limit your "yes" to occasions when you can agree wholeheartedly to do something without reservations. Simply put, if it isn't a "Hell, yes!" then don't do it or be prepared to suffer the consequences.

The reason your energetic boundaries are so important is simply this. It is a fact of life that there will always be more things to do than the energy available to do them, so you need to choose wisely. It is okay to give yourself permission to stop! Create some space, sit yourself down and find out who you are and what you want from your life. Get clear. Define your boundaries. There is a quiet unspoken confidence that comes from having your energy in balance. After all, balanced energy allows us to express our truth and it is this quality that makes us reliable friends, great parents and successful entrepreneurs.

- *Find some space, breathe deeply and allow yourself to meditate on your truth*
- *Allow whatever is true for you to rise to the surface. Listen with your whole body*
- *Allow your truth to resonate at a cellular level*
- *What boundaries do you need to put into place? What boundaries do you want to put in place?*
- *Take notice of what you know*

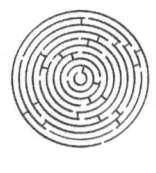

Day 9
Be yourself

The challenge is to be yourself in a world that is
trying to make you into everyone else.

There are many people out there in the world who seem to love complaining. Nothing is ever right for them and their lives seem to lurch from one drama to the next. We all know these people and there may have been times in your life (there certainly was in mine), where you did the same?

My work as a coach has led me to work with a number of these individuals and to gain a respect for how challenging it can be to transform who you think you are at an identity level. *The fear of doing this was always far greater than the actual steps to change.* I found that the difference that made all the difference was always working with and connecting to my client's energy. How can you be yourself when you don't think you like or even know who you are? It takes guts to turn your attention away from what you think is wrong with you, others or your work environment - to shift your energy away from complaints to contribution. It takes daring to become focused on dreams instead of dilemmas. You may become concerned that if you don't ponder on your shortcomings (or those of others) something bad will happen. You maybe so used to living with your problems that the thought of leaving them behind leaves you cold. Don't worry, you're not alone. It doesn't have to be this way.

Once you begin to *raise your awareness* and understand about your energy *you will gain clarity* and that alone puts you into a position of choice. *You can then choose the energy in any given moment that will serve you best.*

For now though, I want you to know that you have everything you need to function perfectly on your energetic journey; nothing has been left out. *There is nothing wrong with you, and there never has been.* I say this, no matter what has happened to you in your life.

Please let that sink in for a minute. Let the words enter your body and move through your center to your heart. Repeat them again. Say them aloud. Allowing this message into your consciousness - this might just allow you to relax, even if for just a moment, to allow your stomach to untie its knots. This is because at the centre of all of us there is a worry, however small, that something is wrong with us, hidden deep down inside, and if we are not careful we will be found out.

Whatever you have gone through in life or are yet to go through, your experiences are the natural consequences of being a human being. How do I know? It's true about me and about everyone I have ever coached, or met - I know it is true about everyone, whether they know it or not. What may also be true for you is that you haven't yet learned to use your energy to bring you what you want from life. To do this, you don't need to change who you are, or even what you think. There is no need for an extreme makeover! The only thing you need to do is to learn to bring forward what is already within you forward, so you can be yourself and live the life you were meant to live.

- *Find a piece of card, one you can carry around in your wallet or pocket, and write onto it... "Nevertheless, I am willing".*
- *Carry this with you for the next few days. Whenever you feel stuck or when you need to make a decision - hold up those words and say them out loud. "Nevertheless, I am willing".*
- *Notice what happens to your energy.*

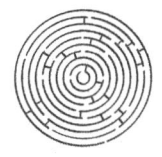

Day 10
Inner voices

The voice in your head is not the voice of God,
it only sounds like it thinks it is.
- Anon

Most of us live disconnected from our true self, we go within and find a crowd of inner voices all battling for attention. In order to grow we need to explore inwardly and outwardly to find the clues to our true self and to begin to notice our calling. I have no idea, for example, where your true path may lie - *but you do*. I know this because I've been privileged to guide many people into their energy awareness and find purpose in their lives. Every single person knows exactly what set of conditions will allow them to fulfill their potential while creating the greatest positive impact on the world. *You are no different.* As you begin to reconnect with what matters most to you and be yourself you may find that you have put other people in charge of charting your course through life, that you are living a life *you feel you "should"*. If this is you, don't worry, personal growth leads us to realizations which can sometimes challenge us at our very core.

Our socialization patterns from early childhood mean we are all shaped by those around us, cultural norms and others' expectations. As a consequence, we learn that our very survival can depend on our ability to please others. This can be a hard habit to break! Your socialized self contains your ego identity and it is this part of you that acts as your self protection. This is the small voice you may hear inside yourself that tries to keep you safe. It wants to protect you from harm and keep you *within your comfort zone*. It likes to protect you from your true self that yearns to be free! The ego is NOT the voice of your intuition or your true self. Thank it, for its concern for you and its protective role, then shift your attention to your true self and pay attention to what really matters deep within. Only then will you be in a position to consciously choose what's next.

You are likely to have other voices within too. Take some time and get to know them. Begin a dialogue with each voice you find and discover what the positive intention is behind their inner role. Once you begin to understand the purpose of each voice you can then decide if the voice is a help or hindrance. You can then thank the voice for its message yet leave yourself conscious to make your own decision about what you will do going forward.

- *Light a candle and sit quietly with yourself*
- *Relax into your breathing and begin to breathe more deeply*
- *Notice the many different voices which lie within. Ask them to come forward one by one. Find out about their role within, what is their intention? Do you have a symbol or name you can give to each voice?*
- *Enter into a dialogue with each voice. Get to know the voice and what message it has for you*
- *Breathe in and appreciate each of your voices*
- *Breathe out and let them know you are always available to listen to the messages they have for you*
- *Relax and know as you develop your inner understanding, you will be free to make your own conscious choices about which voices support you in your life and which sabotage you*

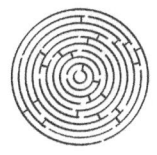

Day 11
Space in between

Out beyond the ideas of right and wrong
there is a field. I will meet you there.
- Rumi

Always leave a little space in your life, you never know what you may need it for. *So many of us fill our lives with stuff and nonsense,* we lunge from one unconscious thing to another and forget to leave some critical time for ourselves along the way. We are so busy dealing with the needs of others, we can forget that we have needs to. We need to take time to pause, to reconnect to what matters most in the space that lies between ourselves and the world. Space is where we notice the limitations that may be holding us tightly in certain areas of our life. It reminds us that where there is space, there is choice and it encourages us to explore a different way of being in the world.

You need space for renewal, for rest and relaxation. Tension in your body can have far reaching and profound effects on your energy and your physical health. Our thoughts, feelings, sensations and actions are threaded together by our energetic network. Physical sensations or muscular activations accompany every thought and emotion. When you can find the space to get out of your head and drop into your body you will begin to notice the messages from your body. You will know if your body needs attention in certain areas. When you are tense or you find that your body is protesting with occurrences of illnesses or injuries it is time to take action. If you are like most of us you will not be able to relax away all of your muscular tension which is when you need to get the help of a specialist and book yourself a much needed massage. Due to the stress of life these days we all have areas of chronic muscular contraction which is beyond the reach of our own inner relaxation techniques. Massage will help you to release. It will actually open up more space within your physical body for the energy to flow.

Space is exciting, it is where the magic happens in your life. When you leave a little space a whole world of possibility opens up to you. Don't forget to book yourself some time out of your regular routine. You can do everything or nothing with this time - *the choice is yours; no-one else's.* This is your time to do with it what you will. Don't allow your entire day to be given away, because days turn into weeks, weeks into months and months into years and before you know it the kids are grown and you've *forgotten to live your life your way*. If you are really unfortunate you may have forgotten to live at all. Be bold, step outside the normal spaces you find yourself within and claim some space back just for yourself!

- *Sit comfortably, breathe deeply and begin to notice your shape*
- *Breathe in and notice where your body feels tense.*
- *As you breathe out allow your muscles to relax. Feel how good it is to release the tension you have been carrying in that spot*
- *Check in with the following areas which are common areas to hold tension in the body: forehead, scalp, teeth and jaw, neck, shoulders, forearms, hands, sphincters, calves and feet. Breathe the tension away.*
- *Sit up a little straighter and allow more space into your spine. Stand up and stretch your body allowing more space within.*
- *As you go through your day today - stay alert to the tension within your body and create more space wherever you can*

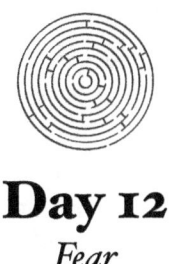

Day 12
Fear

Only when we are no longer afraid do we begin to live.
- Dorothy Thompson

In a very real sense, the surging water in an ocean does not move, it allows the energy to move through it. It is in the same way that the energy of fear moves through our culture. Some experience it as a light and somewhat unpleasant breeze, constantly in the background of their awareness and easy to tolerate. Meanwhile others are destroyed by it, as if by a hurricane. Nobody is untouched. Fear is around us and within us and whilst most of us, in the West at least, do not face mortal danger on a daily basis, we often live as though we do. *We live in fear and call it stress.*

Fear is such a general term it can cover many things. Every day my work as a coach brings me into contact with people who are afraid, anxious or simply worrying. Fear can be such a stifling experience it can make it difficult for us to breathe or it can be a low grade condition, that we become habituated to and get used to living alongside.

Fear is not always negative. Overwhelming fear which you experience in a potentially violent situation is actually energizing, a primal response which encourages you to fight or flight. It is unmistakeable and difficult to ignore. Interestingly when fear is in low grade form at the level of worry, it can be the most pervasive and can drain your energy without you ever realizing it. Fear can steal your aliveness. So what is your fear? Time to get to know your fears. Once you uncover their influences on your life you will come to realize that *you* are so much more than you are fearful of.

If you want to live a seriously fulfilling life then you may as well get used to your fears. In this context *when you feel fear, you know that you are approaching your learning edge* as you continue to stretch and grow. If there is no fear present then you are within your comfort zone and your learning is some distance away. After many years of coaching people through their fear and also facing a number of my own, I know that the only way to get rid of your fear is to move through it, and that usually means facing your fear head on and then stepping directly into it. I have also learned that pushing through fear is far less frightening than living with the underlying fear that comes from a feeling of helplessness. Actually going out and doing whatever it is you are most fearful of usually brings relief. I have found this to really make all the difference as it brings a sense of *empowerment*, a real sense of *accomplishment* that if you can face your fears, what is there now to be afraid of?

Once you can join the dots and make this realization for yourself, that fear itself holds no fear for you, perhaps it is at this point where we actually give ourselves permission to throw off our limitations and *really* begin to live.

- *Center yourself and breathe steadily. As you slow your breathing allow yourself to drop within and your fears to bubble up to the surface*
- *Notice without judgement what you are fearful of*
- *Sit quietly and bring to mind one thread of your fears that you have recently unraveled. Explore how you moved through your fear, notice the emotions that aroused as you did so*
- *Begin to understand your relationship with fear*
- *Allow and accept your fears, invite them into your heart energy*
- *Know that your fears today are not the same as last year, your fears move on as you learn and grow. They give you positive energy to build momentum and become more in your life. Whatever your fears are today, these too will pass.*

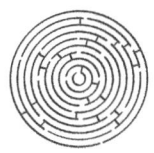

Day 13
Remembering to breathe

When you remember to breathe the rest usually follows

Breath is energy and energy is life. You can affect the way that you feel by becoming conscious of your breathing. Think about those times when you have been anxious, angry or upset in any way; if you do no more than focus on your breathing, feel and follow it, you will have found yourself becoming calmer and less disturbed. You don't have to do anything else, becoming aware of your breathing is all you need to do. It is the first step into presence with your energy.

During every moment of your life, this natural ebb and flow is an essential part of your being. Wherever and however you are sitting or reclining right now, *notice yourself breathe*. Don't try to change anything, just let your breath flow. Feel the *physical sensation* of air coming in through your nose and flowing down into your lungs, then follow it as it flows back out again. What does the air feel like? Does it have a distinctive taste or smell? What is your rhythm of breathing? How long do you inhale before you begin to exhale? Can you feel the air as it passes through your nose, your lips, your teeth? Let your conscious mind unite with your breathing. Notice whether you sometimes hold your breath. Take a few minutes now to do nothing but become conscious of your breathing.

After a while you may realize that you want to change something about your breathing. Perhaps you'd like to breathe more deeply, or slow your breathing, or make some other alteration. Go ahead. Don't force anything, just allow your breathing to move in an easy, natural way. You can let your awareness of breathing carry you into a state of deep relaxation. *It is here in this timeless moment that you will find that there is nowhere to go and nothing to do.* Just be. Let go of all your business, your tension and anything else which might be blocking your energy flow. If your eyes have been open, close them and float into your inner sanctuary, free from worries or concerns. All you have to do is simply breathe, in and out, in and out.

Know that you carry this personal space, this inner sanctuary with you in your daily life. It is there for you as a resting place to return to whenever you wish. All you need to do to get there is to sustain your awareness of breathing in and breathing out and everything else in your life will follow in its own rhythm and right timing.

- *At some point during the busyness of your day today, pause and visit your inner sanctuary.*
- *No matter what is going on around you... breathe.*
- *Breathe like a fallen leaf and think of nothing*
- *Breathe and let your heart and mind be carried , however briefly to the spirit you cannot quite see*
- *Breathe and simply be*
- *Just breathe...*

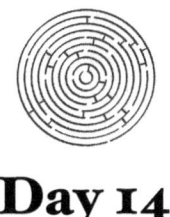

Day 14
Trust

He who does not trust enough will not be trusted.
- Lao-Tzu

In today's world, trust can be a challenging thing to find in our daily lives. How you relate to the world depends in part on how much you trust or mistrust yourself and others. Three recurring threads of advice can be found in both East and West literature: be careful about whom and when you trust; trust when you can; and always behave in a way that deserves the trust of others. Ultimately it is our ability to relax into life that reflects our willingness to trust.

Trust has far reaching consequences; you can cultivate your ability to trust, and your capacity to know when not to trust. As we all know, when you trust, you are letting yourself be vulnerable to the reality or unreality of another person's message as they express it. You are taking a risk that might lead you to swim deeper into an ocean of possibility and love, or plunge you deeply into a snake pit of pain and miscalculations. You may get what you want or not, you might also run into unanticipated consequences. The challenge is that the outcome you receive depends at least in part on what others say and do, of which there are no guarantees and of course you have no control.

Throughout life, we are all continuously learning about trust. Our experiences shape our reality. If you've lived through many broken promises and commitments, you may expect someone, or even people in general, not to come through for you. *Distrust grows in the raw pain of disappointment.* But whatever your history, at a certain point in your life, *who you are becoming is your own doing.* Trust is a feeling that lies deep within you. You are the source of your perception of trust, or your lack of it. Either you believe in someone or you don't. Maybe you believe in your relationship, the future, whatever it is that you find your heart holds dear with hope and faith, or you don't. These are your feelings and you can't blame anyone else for them, they belong to you and they have taken root inside your mind. Just know you can let your past inform you without being chained to it.

Trust increases in our relationships when we become aligned in our energy. When our words and actions communicate the same message. When we live our lives from the center of our soul and we become real and authentic in our own resonant energy. We all know when someone is sending out mixed signals, the contradictions that alert our intuition that something is out of whack. When you hear a mixed message it can be challenging to trust what you hear so don't add to the confusion. Ensure you always speak your truth and show up whole in your energy knowing without exception that you are a person who can be trusted.

- *Take several deep breaths and relax*
- *First consider your physical energy, the physical responses which arise when you consider the concept of trust… what sensations arise for you?*
- *Secondly, your emotional energy, what are you feeling?*
- *Thirdly, your mental energy, what are your thoughts? What do you imagine might happen around trust for you, what ideas surface?*
- *Finally, your spiritual energy, is your inner spirit delighted or fearful? Do you feel energized or drained around your ideas of trust*
- *Notice your energy. Listen to your different messages.*
- *Meditate on your responses.*

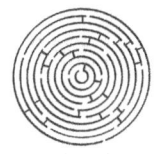

Day 15
Feeling safe and secure

I can lose all my possessions tomorrow,
but I cannot lose who I am

Most things in life are *impermanent* as any Buddhist will tell you. Circumstances arise and then they pass away. Uncertainty is part of life's reality. Much of our struggle with life comes from wanting things that are changing to continue as they were or wanting things to change that are not doing so quickly enough. Our ability to feel safe and secure, to end our suffering in this place is strengthened by our ability to accept, to go with the flow of our lives not against it and dare I say it? Even enjoy, the reality in which we live now.

When you hear the words safe and secure... what comes to mind? You might think of protection in the form of locks, fences, police and soldiers. Or you might bring to mind a partner, friend or family member who truly loves you unconditionally. Such thoughts can tell you something about your own associations and what triggers your feeling of security or insecurity.

However, your feelings of safety are not only confined to circumstances outside of yourself, it is ultimately the way you feel about yourself internally which will drive your behaviors and can end up running you. When someone feels insecure, this can interfere with their energy and their life in many different ways. For example, it is rare for an insecure woman to feel beautiful. It is challenging for a jealous husband to love or trust completely. When insecurity takes the form of a chronic feeling where your physical or emotional survival is threatened, it can lead to acting in desperate ways, cruelty or even violence that ignore's other people's needs and feelings.

Insecurity also affects how others act towards you. It tends to lead to attack and defend interactions with others. When you can develop your ability to feel more secure in yourself, when you find that place of inner safety that lies deep within, you become grounded in your energy. Your energy responds by giving you a strong foundation from which to live your life. You become better able to communicate from a strong, centered inner place where you can get your needs met from the inside out, even in challenging situations. You realize that there is *no need to defend yourself* from others and from your life. You let go and learn to accept impermanence and insecurity, finding that the more you become aware in your energy the more you contribute to your own sense of personal empowerment.

- *Breathe deeply and release into the present moment*
- *Feel into your feelings of safety and security*
- *Are there feelings of insecurity you need to move through you? Allow.*
- *Check in with yourself in this moment, right now*
- *Know that you are safe and secure - all is well with the world*
- *Breathe, you are okay*
- *Breathe in feelings of safety and breathe out any feelings of insecurity*
- *Let go and breathe...*

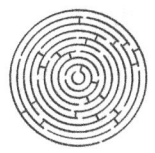

Day 16
Getting out of your head

*If you want to know what your thoughts were like yesterday,
check how your body feels today*

Imagine having a relationship with your body that is *a collaborative partnership*, one in which you and your body are working towards the same goals so that you can show up with the necessary vitality to live your life in a way of your choosing. Let's see if we can set up the foundation for this with the following thought experiment.

Imagine you realize that you and your body are not communicating very well, in fact you are constantly bumping into each other, both fighting for attention and not listening to each other. In short you are just not getting along. It is time to send you and your body for therapy! Yes you need a couples counsellor to help you both out!

Now imagine that you find yourself and your body sitting next to each other on a couch in the counsellors office. The counsellor turns to you first and asks what your complaints are about your body. You take a few minutes to tell her everything. Next the counsellor turns to your body and asks "What are your complaints about this person?". What would your body say about you? What does your body want you to do differently? What messages is your body constantly sending you that you refuse to listen to? How does your body really feel about you?

If you are like most of us maybe some of my body's complaints will resonate with you:
"She never gives me enough rest"
"She looks after everyone else and forgets all about me"

"She never feeds me good quality food, at the right time - she's always rushing around"

"She is always comparing me to someone else who she thinks looks much better than me"

"If I get the slightest pimple she looks at me with disgust"

"She never listens to me, until its too late and I am forced to send her a sledgehammer of pain or an illness"

"This woman never stops! At this rate she'll wear me out in no time"

"She never thanks me for everything I do for her - she only notices when something goes wrong"

If you were in a personal relationship with someone who treated you this way, how long would you want to remain in it? Your body is here to serve you. It has been your partner since the moment you came into physical reality. It is here with you until you leave. You can't do or be anything without it. *Your body loves you.* Yes, really.

Perhaps now is the time for you to shift the focus of your attention away from the complaints you have about your body to the reality that your body is your best friend. Consider for a moment what that means to you, how exactly would you treat your best friend?

- *Sit quietly and allow yourself to drop deep inside your body*
- *Your body is constantly talking to you, but are you listening?*
- *Listen to the messages your body wants you to hear*
- *Breathe slowly and acknowledge what you need to hear*
- *Breathe deeply and commit to move your heart in that direction*
- *Finally, thank your body, appreciate it for everything it does for you on a daily basis*
- *Be at peace within, feeling at home in your own skin*

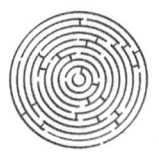

Day 17
Not knowing

It may be when we no longer know what to do
we have come to our real work,
and that when we no longer know which way to go,
we have begun our real journey.
- Wendell Berry

Is "not knowing" an obstacle in your life or a vehicle for your own evolution? You decide. We all get to this place sometimes when we just don't know what to do, think or feel anymore. I have learned to get excited when I reach this place of confusion, or even when my clients do. I know it is this place of not knowing which invites us into a deeper level of exploration with ourselves. It encourages us to go within and to confront and remain open to that which we do not yet know. To complicate the situation *not all of the dimensions of our not knowing are conscious.* We may feel the prodding of instincts, the nudge of our intuition, messages from our unconscious mind without really knowing where they are coming from. This is especially true of things we want to avoid knowing. This is when our not knowing acts to shield us from our pain, to protect us from that which we are not yet ready to know.

I remember when in the depths of my pain how vulnerable I felt. It was because I was beginning what was an *impossible healing journey* without knowing if I would ever recover anything, let alone my health and my life. I didn't know if I was stupid to go against all medical opinion. I ignored the pleadings from close friends and family to listen to the doctors and I chartered my own course, knowing without really knowing that it was somehow inevitable for me to choose this path. Looking back others have said I was courageous. I wonder, because *it felt more like desperation at the time; desperation for even trying.* Back then there was much more that I didn't know than what I knew. Everything I knew I didn't want to know. I found solace in the not knowing. It was my refuge from the pain. I recall the painful paradox of wanting to know how it would all end before I took my first step on the road to recovery and yet I also didn't want to know, as everyone told me what I didn't want to hear. I yearned for the safety and security that comes from knowing I would survive yet it remained elusive. I became broken of all knowing and in this tired and dizzied state, I could see that it didn't really matter whether I knew or not, that knowing and not knowing is no different. It was what I *believed* that would make all the difference. All my fear of not knowing disappeared as I realized only I could determine the outcome for myself. Only I had the power to inform my knowing as within the energy field we are already a part of where we are going. So from that moment I *knew*.

Not knowing brings confusion and confusion is a cauldron for your creativity. It is an escape from a well-ordered world where you may be fooled into believing that in your knowing you have not only clarity but also control. Not knowing is an opportunity for exploration. It can catapult you into a dramatically different way of looking at yourself and the world. You never know, like me, it might just save your life.

- *This is a walking meditation. Center yourself, walk in rhythm with your breathing*
- *Begin to explore what is around you - the simplicity of the leaves on the trees, the air you breathe, other people you meet, the warmth of the sun*
- *Explore your sense of knowing and how it makes you feel*
- *Consider how you know when you put one foot in front of the other the ground will come to support you in your forward movement*
- *Explore your sense of not knowing and how it makes you feel*
- *Consider how your sense of not knowing impacts you and release whatever doesn't support you*

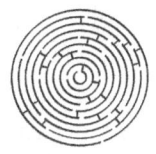

Day 18
Rest and renewal

We are not machines we are human biological systems designed to pulse between activity and rest.

We all know that energy comes from diet, sleep and exercise. But we're also influenced by the extensive network of energy fields which are undetectable to our five senses. For instance, there is gravity, the force of attraction which pulls everything towards the earth's centre, holding us to the ground. Or magnetic fields which attract and repel metals and metallic substances. In a similar way there is an energy field emanating from everything we encounter within our lives and our response to these different frequencies is manifested in our own unique energy levels.

You need to become aware of your energy to know what drains and what revitalizes you. You don't want to join the many folks who unconsciously leak energy wherever they go. I understand how brutally challenging it can be to try to manage your energy. For many years I worked as a consultant, traveling far and wide to serve clients, then arriving home drained and zombie-like after a long day or even week on the road. Oh yes, I forgot to mention I was a single mother to two very vibrant, young girls at the time too. Thankfully, I has some amazing friends who helped me with childcare. Exhausted, I was fearful of declining offers for work as I wanted to secure our financial future. So, I'd accept work and then pay the price at evenings and weekends. Once I had rested though, I was off again never stopping to consider the toll it was having on my body. Even though somewhere deep within I knew better, I was fighting a losing battle trying to honor my body's rhythms.

Finally, the Universe had other plans, sending me a medical injury so severe that I had no choice but to change. I was bed-ridden for over 2 years, registered as disabled by the medical profession and told I would never recover. It was time for me to get to know my body, to take responsibility for my own health and begin to heal myself. It is this healing journey which has given me a *deep appreciation* of my energy and rebuilt my relationship with my physical body.

Maybe you are like me? When I had energy, I assumed I would always have it. I haven't sailed through life either - I walk, run, crawl, fall and pick myself back up. I keep going. There never seemed to be any other choice. But now I find with every challenge I become wiser, somehow freer in myself, and I know how to revitalize my energy to bring myself back to center. Now that I have regained my energy I am so grateful and feel utterly reborn. Whether you reach *a crisis point* which brings you to your knees like mine, or you merely realize you are well on your way to one, you need to treat your energy with respect. *You need to experience how mind blowing it can feel to move fully into flow,* running freely on full capacity and how this involves being as well as doing. Your energy is more mystical and more powerful than you have ever imagined. The truth is you can choose to move to breakthrough with your energy before your body feels it is time to breakdown.

You deserve to live the life you were meant to live and you deserve to have the energy to do it. It is time to listen to your energy and balance your activity with adequate periods of rest and renewal.

- *For today notice what drains your energy and what re-energizes you*
- *Consider how you can shape your day to ensure you have balance between the two*
- *Reclaim your lunch - take some time away from your desk, stop the doing and concentrate on simply being (if only for a few minutes)*
- *Take a break every 3 hours and spend 5 minutes walking, chatting or listening to music (or anything which will invigorate your energy)*

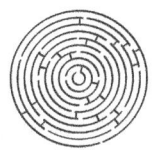

Day 19
The confidence to create

Some people say they haven't found themselves.
But the self is not something one finds,
it is something one creates.
- Thomas Szasz

The Renaissance was a remarkable period in history which emerged from a time of plague, cultural decay and thousands of years of oppressive rule by different Kings and Queens. *Within the span of a single generation* Leonardo, Michelangelo and Raphael produced exceptional works of art, Luther rebelled against the Catholic Church and Columbus discovered the New World amongst other things. Throughout Europe people threw off the chains of tradition and developed a passion for creativity that had long been discouraged. The energy of the time was expansive, energetic and creative.

You can stimulate the same energy in your life too. You can stop using your emotional and mental energy in ways that sabotage your ability to think clearly, feel appropriately and act effectively. You can become aware of your own unique energy system. *Let go* of the habits that are draining your energy whilst your physical body is still strong and healthy and make that energy available for more constructive purposes. When your sense of self is ready for a facelift, you can break out of your time worn patterns of thinking and acting and undergo your own personal renaissance. You can go within and *find the confidence to re-create yourself* and design the life you want to lead.

Creative ideas are not just for artists, you can be creative in many different aspects of your life. Once you can acknowledge the many sides of creativity you open the door to finding your own forms of creative expression. You can enhance your creativity by coming fully into the present moment, by flexibility in thinking and by being open to your imagination. Once you begin to look at and modify your old ways of encountering the world, opportunities for you to become more resourceful open up before you.

Some people are afraid to be creative because they fear other people's criticisms. If I've learned anything whilst traveling my path it is simply this; allow your creativity to express what you are passionate about and don't worry about what others say. Much of the value in creating comes with the energy boost it brings to you. So find your passion and create from that place and notice what happens to your energy!

- *Shift into your center and make yourself comfortable*
- *Scan your consciousness for any creative yearning that you have that has not yet been fulfilled*
- *Uncover a meaningful creative desire*
- *Watch your thoughts here, are you supporting your energy or draining it? Are you getting in your own way?*
- *Examine your life from different points of view - how can you embrace more creativity in your daily life?*
- *Ask your intuition how you might best use your creativity*
- *Listen and take notice. Go out and enjoy a creative day!*

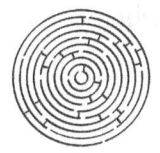

Day 20
Coming home

We shall not cease from exploration
And the end of our exploring
Is to arrive as the start
And to know it for the first time.
- T. S. Eliot

You are more strong and powerful than you realize. You are resourceful, creative, independent, sensitive and intuitive and when you bring all these qualities together you feel confident, alive, energetic, successful, assertive and empowered. You are made up of more than just your physical body, *you are energy in action*. You have highly developed energetic bodies which communicate to others the messages of your mind, body, spirit and emotions. Your energetic power is within you - come home and reconnect to this energy, and you will find that you radiate a smile from the inside out! Everything you need to be happy is inside of you, you can radiate from within.

Coming home can mean more than just coming home to yourself - who else in your life do you need to come home to? Where is your home base? That place where you feel you belong, where you feel comfortable, secure, loved and trusted. It is the foundation from which you live your life. Knowing where your base is can give you stability when all around you seems to be moving in the wrong direction. It gives you your roots, your stability to go out into the frenetic pace of the world and find a way to make a difference. When you find yourself feeling lost, touching base can be a real joy. It can remind you that you have a place where you are accepted no matter what, it can give you back some perspective on what is really important in your life. And when you do it, you will wonder why you don't do it more often.

Never be too busy for your family. It is so easy in today's fast paced life to ignore the people who are closest to us - I know because I am as guilty as you! It might be our children, our parents, our spouse, our siblings or our best friend but I can guarantee there will be someone who you would like to spend more time with, someone that you just haven't managed to find the time to call to just find out simply how they are, or to dedicate some time just for them, without distractions. Unforgivable. Don't settle for living with the guilt - do something about it now. Plan a time when you can put everything down and give them your full attention. One day they might not be there, then it will be too late. So make time for the people who matter today.

- *Sit quietly and reconnect with your home base that lies deep within you*
- *Bring to mind those who you may have been neglecting in your life. Meditate on the love you carry for those dear to your heart*
- *Breathe deeply and allow yourself to come home to that love and sense how it wants to express itself now*
- *Call out to the Universe with your love. Imagine yourself sending out an energetic stream of love to those on your mind*
- *Do not defer the expression. Do not push it back down. Act today. Go home.*

Recorded by the author, '**An Energetic Journey**' is a free Guided Meditation that accompanies this book.

For your copy, go to: **https://rebrand.ly/AEA-Meditation**

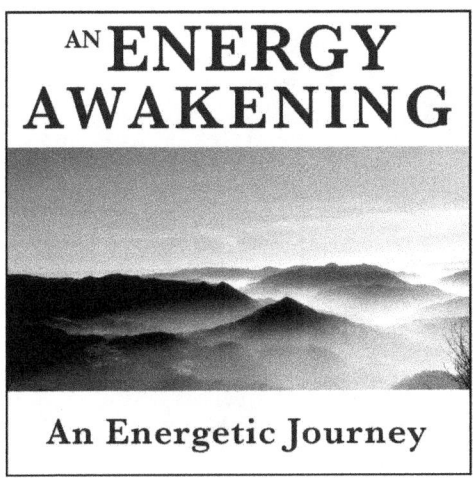

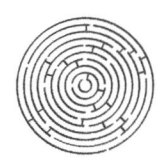

Part Two: Healing the Past

Although the world is full of suffering it is also full of the overcoming of it.

– Helen Keller

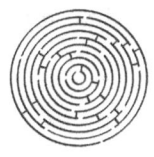

Day 21
Legacies from the past

"The past is a foreign country, they do things differently there"
- L.P. Hartley

The past may be who you were at one point in time, but it does not have to be who you are today. *There is no need for you to continuously carry the legacies of the past along for the ride.* The ways that we think, feel and behave create the quality of our lives. If you think that you are not good enough, you will feel inadequate and lack confidence. Life will be challenging and you are likely to become a passive victim constantly trying to survive everything that life throws your way. It doesn't have to be this way!

Chances are you picked up these beliefs about yourself when you were very young, so it can be interesting to take a step back and consider the bigger picture. Ask yourself, not just why you feel this way but also how it got to be like that. Listen to your intuitive response. Now you have choice. *Step out of the past and into the present moment.* Check in with yourself. When you stop the old patterns of your past and stop worrying about the future, you are able to enter into the present moment and you will find YOU ARE OKAY! Right now in this moment, it is rare to find that you are threatened. Coming out of the past and living in the now is the simplest way of letting go and being fully present in your life.

Your habits can also shape your current reality. We fill our days with habitual behavior, we just do what we do, day in and day out. When someone challenges us we say "It's just me, it's who I am"... really? Most of us are better at looking after everyone else than we are at looking out for ourselves. It is time for a change. Look after yourself. If you don't who will?

Take care of your physical energy by eating well, sleeping more and exercising often.

Take care of your emotional energy by acknowledging and accepting how you feel about things; let the river of your emotions move through you.

Take care of your mental energy by giving yourself downtime, find the space within your mind and get present.

Take care of your spiritual energy by knowing what is really important to you by connecting and living from your soul.

- *Center yourself and with each breath put aside the things you think should be*
- *Breathe deeply and with each breath put down the negative things you are carrying from your past*
- *Breathe in and with each breath put aside who you think you are*
- *Breathe out and let go of anything which is not serving you well*
- *Sit in the center of your being without these things and know that you are as beautiful as a mountain spring. You are enough. It is time to let go.*
- *Breathe and release*

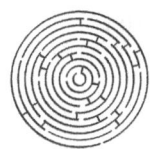

Day 22
Courage

Life shrinks or expands in direct proportion to one's courage.
- Anais Nin

Like many of us, I seem to be continuously challenged to have the courage to step fully into my life and *be real*. To show up whole. To be connected to the very deepest parts of me and yet still respond to the presence in every moment. To be uniquely and independently me. Sometimes when I catch a glimpse of the flow of my life it is easy. I feel grounded, open and can shoot the breeze, incredibly comfortable with who I am. Other times... it's not so easy. No matter how much I reach out from my core there remain parts of me that step back. When this happens, I have noticed that there is one critical decision I face that makes all the difference.

At the threshold of your *true independence* is the same decision which offers you the key to your personal liberation and happiness. It takes courage, but the benefits are well worth it. In psychological terms it is often highlighted as a major factor in psychological maturity, and yet I have met many adults who have yet to embrace this concept. It literally makes the difference between success and failure. So ask yourself :
"*Are you ready to accept complete responsibility for who you are and for everything that you become?* Are you ready to accept complete responsibility for your business and its success or failure?"

We are talking complete responsibility, no excuses, no blame, no judgements, just 100% responsibility. You must accept without reservation that you are *where you are and what you are, because of yourself. If you want things to change, you must change first.* Your thinking determines your attitude and your behavior and they in turn largely determine the quality of your life. Since you are always free to choose the content of your conscious mind, you are always fully responsible for what you think. You can dream big dreams, learn how to control your thinking and improve your self-concept and performance, BUT *it won't give you any lasting benefit until you embrace personal responsibility.*

You know it is time to take full responsibility when you realize that everything you will ever become is completely up to you - no-one else is going to do it for you. Now forgive me, I know you know this at some level logically speaking, but do you *really* know it? *Does it resonate within your energy?* The acceptance of complete responsibility means giving up on all of your excuses. It is not easy. It is one of the hardest things you will ever attempt. It is like making a parachute jump for the first time - scary and exhilarating. When you let go of all your excuses, as when you leap out of a plane, you suddenly feel completely alone and extremely vulnerable. However, within a few moments you start to feel a rush of excitement, your heart starts pounding faster and you feel free and happy.

Self-responsibility is the core quality of the fully mature, fully functioning, self-actualizing individual. To live a life worth living you need to take both the credit and the blame for everything that happens to you. You need to have a strong sense of internal accountability which extends to all your relationships and your business life. Research suggests that there is a direct relationship between how much responsibility you are willing to accept for results both positive and negative AND your income, your health, your status and your level of success.

- *Center yourself and meditate on how you are showing up to your world*
- *Breathe slowly and connect to your courage*
- *Know from this moment on you will take 100% responsibility for your thoughts, your emotions and your actions. You are ready.*

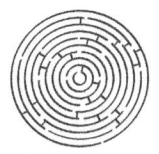

Day 23
In the shadow

We are not to be underestimated.
But the only intelligence on the planet that could ever underestimate us is ourselves
- Jon Kabbat-Zinn

Without light there is no shade. We all have aspects of ourselves which we would rather remain hidden. However, I have noticed that I keep finding myself in situations where I am required to be all of who I am in order to find my way through. It takes both my light and my shade, my strength and my vulnerability for me to show up in a way that enables my life to open before me and evolve. When I don't my life just seems to stall.

When you don't acknowledge your shadow you implicitly give it permission to run your show, and although it may be the last thing on your conscious mind, you sabotage your own plans. e.g. you have a plan but you aren't taking the action steps you need to follow through and reach your goal. *Why would you get in your own way?* Resistance, fear and that small voice inside that never has anything good to say!

There are reasons why you resist what you really want. There are payoffs. It's much easier to keep doing what you already know how to do as it saves you from facing your feelings of fear and limitation. It can be easier to keep dreaming about a better life, hoping that one day, by magic all your cares will be swept away. At least this way you never have to face yourself head on. You will have all come across the saying *"Better the devil you know than the devil you don't"*. Your current circumstances are familiar to you. When you don't take a risk you can make excuses of being responsible or practical. It all seems to make sense rationally, doesn't it?

For those of us committed to exploring our potential, to using our energy to really feel alive, rational doesn't really work. We yearn for something more a higher level of engagement and a sense of adventure and that takes a little more investment.

Invest in yourself by treating yourself as though you count. All of you. Get to know your shadow, and if you prefer, get a coach or therapist to guide you along the way. *People respond to those who show up whole.* Move beyond your resistance. It is time for you to accept all of you and offer everything up to the light. You are more amazing than you currently know!

Try this exercise to help you move past your resistance.

- *Center yourself and ask "How much do I want to stick with my belief that I can't do ... "*
- *Take some time to meditate on any current change you are considering*
- *Consider your perceptions of Loss versus Gain. Make a list of everything you think you will lose or gain from this change. Which list is longer? Which elements of your list are more important? What did you forget?*
- *Make friends with your inner critic. This is the voice of your ego or false self. It can be bad news as your brain believes what you tell it about yourself. It is true that you become what you think, so choose your thoughts wisely. Always ask yourself, "Is that true?".*
- *Focus on your positives and turn your negative thinking into positive statements. e.g. "I'm not good at relationships" can become "I am learning more about relationships and showing signs of improvement.".*
- *Relax and breathe. Allow yourself to know what there is to know about your shadow. Accept whatever comes. Know you are complete. You are whole. Commit to bringing your whole self into your life today.*

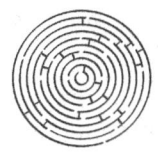

Day 24
Feeling your feelings

The best and most beautiful things in the world
cannot be seen or even touched.
They must be felt with the heart.
- Helen Keller.

What is it that happens to us during our lives which makes us think we need to repress our emotions and that it's not okay to show how we feel? We are human beings and we have emotions. This is normal, repressing our emotions isn't. It is okay to feel your feelings both positive and negative.

It is quite natural, you might say even human, to feel big things deeply and it is okay to let it all show. You don't have to be ashamed of your feelings. I don't care if you are male or female, gay or straight, or any other reason you may come up with why it is alright for others but not for you. I often have clients apologizing for crying during an emotional coaching session. All too often we have learned to contain our true feelings and pretend to the world everything is fine. It is okay to cry, it doesn't mean there is something wrong with you! Pushing your feelings away and repressing your emotions is not a good idea. They just get squashed and will come back to bite you at some point in the future.

The best way to deal with emotions is to let them out, accept you feel this way and *express the emotion fully* (and yes, my clients will tell you I do mean fully!) Then you can get back to living your life. It can often be as simple as that. Too often we become overly concerned of what might happen if we loosen our control of our emotions just a little. If we let them out will we be able to put them back and get on with life? *Unexpressed emotions don't go away.* They have a habit of running you from the inside out, they can get in the way and sabotage your relationships, your happiness and your success. Contrary to popular belief, psychological denial is not a skill worth having.

Once you begin to really feel your feelings you also learn where your true happiness comes from. This is not something you can learn from a book, you really do have to get to know yourself and what makes *you* truly happy. My idea of true happiness wouldn't be the same as yours. *But how do you know when you have true happiness and where does it come from?* Just think about this for a moment, your true happiness is a feeling that you get, right? You might get it when you fall in love, or you buy something amazing for yourself or win the lottery, but it is a feeling nonetheless and all feelings are generated from inside of you. People can get addicted to buying new stuff or gambling just because they like the feeling, without realizing they already have it deep inside. The secret is knowing how to trigger this feeling without anyone or anything else being involved. So take some time out of your day to drop inside, find that positive happiness feeling and live your day today from that place.

- *Find a quiet, still space and enter a meditation with a loved one you feel safe with*
- *Focus on a painful emotion that it has been difficult to hold inside you*
- *Express your emotion as deeply as possible, not necessarily the circumstances of this pain, but the feeling of carrying it, while the other listens in silence*
- *Once you have expressed your pain fully, allowing it to resonate in every cell of your being, allow the listener to offer you comfort. Accept*
- *Sit together in silence, knowing your loved one is there for support, your emotion is released and you can go back lighter to your world*
- *Appreciate and embrace your partner*

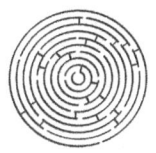

Day 25
The power of optimism

A pessimist sees the difficulty in every opportunity but an optimist
sees the opportunity in every difficulty
- Winston Churchill

What does being an optimist really mean? Does it mean we always *feel* positive? Does it imply we have no concerns for the future? Does it suggest that we will forget our challenges and negative feelings and appear sunny no matter what? The answer to these sensible and enquiring questions is comfortingly, no. *To be optimistic doesn't mean that you have to forget how you are really feeling about something;* you don't have to deny your negative feelings and pretend everything is okay when it is not. Being optimistic is a much deeper notion than walking around feeling happy. It basically relates to your ability to make the best of what you have got, to optimize yourself and your circumstances regardless of what life brings your way.

It seems to some degree, optimism is an inborn trait. Several research studies have found that optimism runs in families, though none of the studies can determine exactly what genetic code or brain chemistry is responsible. But what if you weren't born into the optimistic family, is all hope lost for you? Or is optimism something you can develop like learning to ride a bike? Thankfully *optimism is a skill we can all learn.* Unfortunately, many of us are brought up only too familiar with the negative side of things. We live in a world full of upsetting events and everyday stresses. As children, even those of us who grew up in the most loving of families, were exposed to a startling array of negative experiences as we began to develop our energetic foundation for life. By the time most of us reach adult life, we are usually carrying our own unique baggage filled with our individual rejections, our disappointments and other dense emotional energy which can make the ability to be optimistic yet another thing to add to our self development checklist.

How many times have you heard someone say, "Hey, cheer up!" or "Turn that frown upside-down!"? Unconsciously we all seem to know that optimism is a virtue and that a negative outlook is something to be concerned about. So we instantly feel that if we are not feeling naturally optimistic then there must be something wrong with us. Not so. Optimism is about focusing your energy on the positive without denying the negative. It is about using energy in a sustained way to influence what is controllable and optimizing your opportunities, your performance and your results.

The key is to become aware of your own energy, to know yourself really well on a physical, emotional, mental and even spiritual level. To know what has a negative affect on your energy and to learn to minimize its impact. Once you become more in tune with how you show up to your life, the next step is to generate your energy from within and not let external circumstances dictate your emotional state. No matter what is happening around you, if you can develop your optimistic attitude at the core of your being, you will equip yourself to survive any challenge, any disappointment, any crisis, and any source of upset. After all, every hardship, every seemingly impossible challenge is actually just a brilliant opportunity for you to show how far you can stretch yourself to accomplish your goals.

- *Sit quietly and explore your own unique nature*
- *How do you really feel about yourself and your life?*
- *How do you show up to your relationships? Your career? Your life?*
- *What would others say about your approach to life?*
- *How can you reconnect to your own innate sense of optimism deep within?*
- *What is there for you to learn today?*

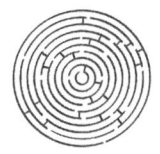

Day 26
Where we've been

Though no-one can go back and make a brand new start,
anyone can start from now
and make a brand new end.
- Anon.

Dwelling on the past is perhaps one of the greatest obstacles to your energy. The more we focus on what happened to us yesterday, especially how unfair and how unpleasant it was, the more we are guaranteed to miss the beauty in our lives. This is true whether what we are thinking about is positive or negative. Not only do we *miss* what is happening in the now but we also *fail* to hear the voice of our intuition, guiding us along our rightful path.

During the depths of my illness, I used to think of myself *as a victim*. When people asked me about my life I would tell them about my pain, which stretched from my childhood through the ending of my first marriage, to my overwhelming medical injury. I was defining myself through all the things that seemed to have gone wrong with my life. It was harrowing and intensely sad, each time I told the story I would relive the negative emotions draining any positive life force out of my body. Healing was not something I even considered whilst in the quagmire of my woe.

Even though my story was true it was a sad restricting story that kept me defined by my own negative experiences. The more I focused on my past the less I connected with who I was today or to where I was going. I was not allowing a new emerging story to take place. I needed to look forward in my life not backwards. The moment I made the decision to let go of this story, I released myself from an incredible burden. It freed me up energetically to discover the new story of who I am today (and also who I want to become tomorrow). This was truly an act of liberation which opened my healing heart allowing me to discover a deeper connection with myself, to realize that I am more than my story and in fact *I can choose the next story for a new chapter of my life*. Our experiences never fully define who we are, they are best used to learn from and then released.

When you let go of your past your present truth emerges. It takes lots of energy to carry your past along with you all of the time. Why not let it go and liberate your energy for more productive uses in your life?

- *Find some space and focus your attention and appreciation on the story of you*
- *Bring it to mind as thoroughly and dramatically as possible - remembering the different people you have told and the different ways you have of telling it*
- *Consider the payoffs for you when telling your story - how does it make you feel?*
- *Decide today to let it go - release your story of you and make space for a new story to emerge. Let go of the past and step into the present. It's time for a new story.*

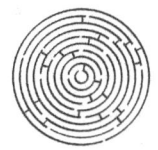

Day 27
When life is hard

When everything seems to be going against you,
remember that the airplane
takes off against the wind, not with it.
- Henry Ford.

Are you ready to move past your struggles and feeling stuck? I know, who's going to say "no"! Perhaps now is the perfect time for you to leverage your personal performance. We are not talking about a small incremental step, it is time for you to completely change the rules of your personal plan and *leap ahead.* You see, many of us ordinarily rely on what is obvious. We stay with the same routines, the same people and even the same habits and behaviors that seemed to have worked okay for us in the past. It is an approach that works well and keeps us safe. *We become very attached to what we know will bring us steady and predictable results.* There is no doubt it enables us some degree of success.

When life is hard this is where many of us go. We stay the same. We choose the patterns of behaviors which *minimize* our risk. We hunker down and wait until the storm has passed before we dare to even consider a different route. We become over-dependent on the strategies and tactics we know and resist the opportunities to try something new because they feel clumsy, unknown and, inevitably, involve more risk. Many of us continue working in this way even when the results are screaming that life has moved on and a different way would bring more effective results. So how can we change this and learn to take the golden opportunity which is available to us when times get tough?

If you want to *accelerate your rate of achievement* then you must actively search out and employ new behaviors.

Get uncomfortable. This is not going to feel easy, especially at first. If you are doing something differently you will be stepping outside of your comfort zone. Prepare yourself for a wild ride. You are going to encounter different things, some of which may prove to be obstacles that block your way. If you're like most of us, your normal reaction will be to hang on tightly, just as you would on the fastest roller coaster ride. *My advice is don't.* I am sure to some of you that may feel counterproductive; it is certainly different. *You are going to have to learn to let go.* Success is achieved through release. If you're feeling a little uneasy then you are at your learning edge - which means you are growing and developing. Get used to this feeling. If you want to be exceptional, you need to keep evolving. *It's time for you to leap off the ledge and grow your wings on the way down.*

STOP trying harder. Sooner or later you are going to reach the point where you can't try any harder. Your enthusiasm will wane and your physical and mental energy will become stretched to its limits. You will reach the point where trying harder and harder starts producing less and less. Time to....

Be brave. Abandon the status quo. Look for a paradoxical move. Brainstorm. Try being illogical. Stop swimming upstream and move into flow. Create some space where you can. Liberate your thinking to begin to try on the idea of doing something else. Focus on possibilities. Move beyond your mental boundaries. Get out of your place of stuckness and move onto the next place.

- *So how are you feeling? What is coming up when you hear these radical ideas to move you forward in times of adversity? Really listen to your inner voice... is it your fears speaking? Or is it your true self?*
- *What is it that you need to surrender to enable you to make a significant shift? Are you getting in your own way? How?*
- *Let your intuition inform you about your leap...*

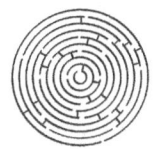

Day 28
The night sky

If we imagine ourselves as being every bit
as huge, deep, mysterious and awe-inspiring
as the night sky, we might begin to appreciate
how complicated we are as individuals,
and how much of who we are is unknown
not only to others but to ourselves.
- Thomas Moore.

In the heart of every person I have ever spoken with I have seen the desire to somehow find true happiness and true fulfilment. Occasionally this desire is stronger than the instinct to survive. As you will know from your own experiences, the search for happiness can take many different paths; for many it is looking for satisfaction in external things... money, career, relationships, food, sex, workouts, designer clothes etc. I don't need to tell you that this approach doesn't work because I know you already know this. but has knowing this changed anything for you?

Usually when we have accomplished some level of success in terms of pleasure and comfort, it is then that we recognize that none of it truly satisfies the deeper command within us. We may find moments of beautiful revelation, and certainly moments of pleasure, yet underneath it all is the *fear* that we will never find permanent or true happiness. Our fear of losing whatever peace or happiness we have causes a tension, a contraction as we constantly try to hold on. This is when we know it is time to begin a different journey to explore the infinite potential which lies within. Going within can be a perilous journey, it is like journeying deep into space (where no man has ever gone before!) deep into our own night sky. It can challenge us, as there is little feedback to know if we are doing it "right" or to satisfy our modern need for stimulation. Modern life offers us a never-ending supply of things and ideas that excite our emotions and desires. You won't find your sense of self nestled amongst fluffy white clouds and green meadows with a neon light flashing above, because *inside is not a place, it's a state of mind.*

Often as you journey within *you are being transformed*, and you may find it hard to tell what if anything, is really happening. While struggling with the pain of your own changes, it can be impossible for you to see the new self you are becoming. It is however, a fascinating journey that will help you to delve into the depths of your unconscious mind in ways that will enrich your daily life. You'll travel through doorways of understanding that will open up new perspectives and possibilities. It will lead you into the inner chambers of your mind where little known sides of yourself remain hidden and you may find things that surprise you, as you begin to develop an appreciation for things you like about yourself. And you'll learn to do a few things or maybe even many, that you've never done before.

The simple truth is we all need a taste of our own night sky, we need to delve into the complexities of being human, of our conscious and subconscious, to enable a greater understanding of ourselves and our lives as they unfold in all their majesty before the ground beneath our feet.

- *This is a night time meditation*
- *Go out after dark and find yourself a place to rest underneath the stars*
- *Sit quietly and go within - notice the depth of your being*
- *Be with whatever you find - if you notice any struggle - just breathe through it*
- *Bless the part of you that is waiting to be uncovered and returned to the world*

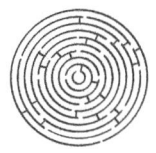

Day 29
When you're feeling stuck

The problem is not that there are problems.
The problem is expecting otherwise and
thinking that having a problem is a problem.
- Theodore Rubin.

Don't get stuck with thoughts that don't move. Once your thinking gets crystallized and rigid you've lost the battle. Once you think you have all the answers, or you get set in your ways, then you may as well give up now, you are already part of history. When you are stuck in your thinking, your energy is blocked and this can trigger many different challenges for you. To get the most out of life, keep your options open and your thinking and your life *flexible*. It might just save your life, literally!

Take a reality check. Don't make assumptions about yourself, your life or even about others. If you assume. then you will think you know something, but the truth is you don't. If you seek the truth you might not like the answers you get, but at least you'll know. *Ask powerful questions.* Questions can give you clarity, they demand answers, and answers require people to engage their mental energy and think things through. *Ask questions of yourself constantly.* Ask why you think you are right or wrong, *why* you are doing certain things and *why* you want what you want. Question yourself powerfully and rigorously. You need it. We all do. *It keeps us from assuming we know what's best for ourselves.*

When you get stuck you fail to see the many different opportunities surrounding you. You close your eyes to the possibilities. You shut down. *You begin to live life as a self-fulfilling prophecy.* Your glass is half full and likely to stay that way. In order to breakthrough, you have to be ready to go the moment an opportunity presents itself or when life throws you a curve ball - and you know that always happens when you least expect it! The second you are offered an opportunity to have an adventure, to change your thinking, to step outside of yourself - *just go for it* and see what happens. I guarantee when you do, it will charge your energy. It can light a fire in your belly that will get you moving, bringing some much needed momentum and to get you unstuck.

If the thought of stepping out scares you, do it anyway! Remember you can always retreat back to your comfort zone of being stuck the second it's over... if you really want to, of course.

- *Go for a walk alone and consider your feeling of being stuck*
- *Look down at your feet and know that movement is a natural part of your being. Check in with yourself... what are you not telling yourself? What do you need to move forward? Really? Is that the truth?*
- *What are you afraid of?*
- *What would you do if you knew you couldn't fail?*
- *Breathe deeply and know at a cellular level you are capable of taking the first step. You don't have to know everything about your journey. You only need to take the first step and allow your journey to unfold before you.*

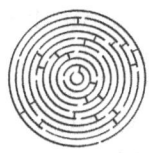

Day 30
Emptiness

It had never occurred to me that feeling empty
might actually be a route to something
deeper and richer within.
- Tony Schwartz

As you read this, simply relax. Empty your mind. Empty yourself. *Go beyond your identity, beyond your thoughts and emotions and see what lies within.* Be and do absolutely nothing. In this process of relaxation, see if any tendencies arise for you to do something. Do you feel the urge to do or make something useful in this moment, to either try to keep this moment with you or to push it away? Do you resist from resting in your *emptiness*?

For most of us thinking of ourselves as empty is a terrifying thought, nobody wants to amount to "nothing at all" in this life. If we are empty perhaps this means we are dispensable and as such will be discarded for something of more value. We think of emptiness as value, of something devoid of life, devoid of energy. If we think we are empty we can develop feelings of worthlessness and at the extreme thoughts of death and destruction can pervade our very being as we develop an inner fear which can be very strong.

Our mental energy defends us against nothingness and we can develop energetic patterns wrapped around our fears. "What does this mean?" your mind may be crying out for attention. Why? It wants to prove that it is *something!* "If I am nothing, how can I do my job? I must be worth something surely...." Let all those frustrated thoughts fall aside and rest in your emptiness. *Do nothing and be empty.* If in this moment, you can actually, willingly. consciously, *simply be nothing at all*, in a flash you might discover the peace that lies deep within. There is *freedom* in emptiness. There is *wisdom* in emptiness.

As a coach I often find that clients come to me to learn new skills, tools and techniques - new ways of being in the world. Many clients are so full, there is no room for anything more. They have to *unlearn* first. Empty out all those thoughts, beliefs and *stuff* which is filling their system and *blocking their energy*. Once they are empty there is plenty of space for new ideas to emerge. In your life you have no need to be concerned when you feel empty. *Empty is good.* Empty creates space and we all know that space is where the magic happens. It allows for your energy to flow. When you find the courage to stay with the emptiness you will experience at least a hint of the boundless peace which lies inside and is always present. If in your emptiness you find a desire to *be* or *do* something else, it is usually time to listen. Stop hiding from the concept of emptiness and experience the wealth that lies within.

- *Sit quietly and simply let yourself breathe*
- *Open your lungs to emptiness and feel the rush of air that naturally moves inwards*
- *Let go of your thoughts*
- *Let go of your emotions*
- *Let go of yourself*
- *Become an empty vessel*
- *Try not to think and also try not to not think*
- *Exhale everything and arrive in your own rhythm at nothing.*

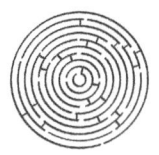

Day 31
Frustration

Frustration is often an edge, not an ending.
- Greg Levoy

I am not sure if it is our human nature that makes change so difficult, but I have found that *we seldom become all of who we are until we are forced to it.* When we become so frustrated with ourselves, others or the circumstances we find ourselves in, we are left with no other choice but to change. So what is this frustration, this emotion, which calls us to become more in our lives?

I have come to the belief that it is our destiny to be opened to our lives, whether we choose this or not. Whether we want to or not, we will, in time find ourselves beyond our edges in a way that may even surprise us. Frustration is merely the guide.

You may think that frustration is an annoying reflex of being human. I agree. No-one likes to be frustrated. It is a product of our expectations. A response to the external and internal pressures which we impose upon ourselves and others. *Where there is no pressure, there is no judgement and no frustration.* We can do ourselves a great disservice by judging where we are in comparison to some final destination. One of the great challenges of living a life where you are continuously striving to be better, is that you are always considering yourself in relation to some imagined landscape of what you are striving for. It is as though wherever we are, it is never enough. We become frustrated with ourselves for being too slow, too fat, too boring, too lazy, too stupid... the list is endless. What will it take for us to move *beyond* our frustration?

Before my medical injury I was extremely driven in my career. I pushed myself greatly. My secret need to achieve excellence made me stretch myself until something within my energy began to rip. It was the unending, relentless way I pushed myself to do more and have more, to put everyone else's needs before my own. I became frustrated as I was caught in a spiral and there never seemed to be enough of anything. I don't believe people bring illnesses upon themselves but I do believe that wherever our energy is weak, it is that part of ourselves which will give way to illness first. Perhaps one of the hardest lessons in life is learning that wherever we find ourselves, however we find ourselves wanting, whatever pain we find in our becoming, *it is all a necessary part of our path*. And whoever we are along the way is *exactly* who we are meant to be doing exactly what we are meant to be doing in that moment.

Frustration can show you a turning point. It can be a gateway to leading a better life. It is your frustration that can call you further into experience than you may be willing to go alone, but it these extra steps that will take you beyond your edge, that ensures you land in the energetic center of what it actually means for you to be wholly and truly alive.

- *Close your eyes and meditate on who you are and who you are becoming*
- *Notice any frustrations which arise as you contemplate your life today*
- *What is the potential turning point for you within your frustration?*
- *What is the message that lies within?*

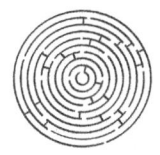

Day 32
Cleaning your wounds

You did what you knew how to do
and when you knew better, you did better.
- Maya Angelou

One of the essential requirements for true spiritual growth and deep personal transformation is coming to peace with pain. I know this because I have lived it, not only in my own life, but by guiding many of my clients through theirs. *No expansion or evolution can take place without change,* and periods of change are not always comfortable. Change involves instability as we dare to question what is familiar and comfortable to us and begin to explore life beyond our comfort zone. As we find ourselves on shifting sands we often perceive this as a painful experience and pain usually leaves its mark.

We all have wounds. I have yet to meet anyone who has not suffered some form of rejection in their life. Becoming familiar with your pain is part of your growth. Since avoiding the pain prevents you from exploring those critical parts of your being beyond your usual self. *Real growth* can only take place when you finally decide to open up to your wounds and deal with the pain.

During the depths of my despair when I was suffering from overwhelming physical pain, and being given pain relief which never seemed to work, it soon became obvious that I had to live *with* my pain. It had become my ever present companion. It would never leave, it would stalk me wherever I went. The most terrifying aspect of this was the prospect that the pain would never end. I was unable to imagine my life beyond the pain, it was almost as though the pain had taken over my life, I had become the pain. I couldn't find the edges of where the pain ended and anything else began. Cleaning my gaping wounds was not an option as I was too busy fighting the pain to see beyond it. The breakthrough came for me when I realized I had a *choice*. I could ground myself and allow the pain to move through me. I knew I was larger than my pain and this empowered me.

When you feel pain simply view it as energy. Start seeing your inner pain as energy passing through your heart, your body and into your consciousness. Then *relax*. If you close around the pain and stop it from passing through, it will stay in you. Trust me, I know this only too well. *Our natural tendency to resist is so counterproductive.* The only way to clean your wounds is to actually *release* and let the energy pass through you. Every time you resist and close, you are *blocking* the pain inside. It's like damning up a river. You are then forced to use your psyche to create a layer of distance between you and your pain. Your wounds turn into scabs, rigid and dry and this can waste a lot of your personal energy.

- *Take some space and ground yourself*
- *Focus on a physical or emotional pain that is within you*
- *As you inhale, accept your pain and allow it to move through your body. Relax*
- *As you exhale release the pain - just let it go*
- *As you repeat this, focus on any moments which are pain free and invite them to expand in your awareness*

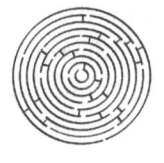

Day 33
After the pain

Give yourself time to heal. Emerge better.

It is incredibly difficult to describe the pleasure that is known once you begin to surface through pain and you find yourself (thankfully!) coming up for air. Hippocrates once said that pleasure is actually the *absence* of pain and anyone who has ever suffered knows this to be true at a deep level. I remember the day in a hospital in the North of England where my physical pain was coupled with an intense emotional pain so intense I thought I would never recover. I was sitting in my doctor's office at the time, following a multitude of tests as she gave me her diagnosis of my medical condition. She told me in no uncertain terms that nothing further could be done for me. It was her professional opinion that I was destined for life in a wheelchair, bedridden and inevitably on huge doses of opiate medication. My disabled status was official and here to stay. She delivered the life crippling message in a tone usually reserved for naughty children and berated me for daring to think that I could begin to lower the doses of my medication. Silly me.

Once I accepted this, which took many tears and more time than I care to remember... I realized there was *nowhere* to run. I understood that what was terrifying about the pain was that it would never end. Life would somehow freeze around the pain in a drug induced haze which would eventually consume any spark of my vitality that remained. I would be lost somewhere deep within, trapped and unable to escape. I would be broken, nothing would exist but the pain.

The breakthrough moment came for me many months later as I was sitting in my wheelchair in a bookstore and my son who by now was a toddler, wandered over with a colorful book for me to read to him. He had picked up Louise Hay's *"You can heal your life"*. This book literally saved me. I knew intimately right then that I had a *choice*. There would be light in my life again, and it would be filled with all the colors of the rainbow - I was ready to get my life back. *The pain of remaining the same was worse than the pain of daring to change.* It was my time to heal. Whether that was a possibility or not was no longer an issue - I knew I had to at least *try*. If nothing else, living with hope was a better place to be.

I also remember that day, not too long ago as I sat on my boat dock in the heat of the Florida sun and realized that I was no longer living a life focused on my pain. I was shocked and surprised to realize I was living beyond the edge of my pain. I had come up for air, I could look up and notice the sun, and it was *shining*. I had been successful. I had healed.

I have noticed that in our despair we often see our pain as something that will never end. In fact we allow this to define us, as though the pain actually consumes our very being and becomes us. In contrast, I know there is a sense of peace for us all to work towards as I am so thankful to be able to share with you that I now know *there is life* after the pain.

- *Find some space and breathe deeply to center yourself*
- *Focus on a physical or emotional pain that is with you*
- *As you inhale consider all that is larger than your pain*
- *As you exhale release the pain into the environment around you that is pain free*
- *Imagine the air beyond your pain and relax into that space*

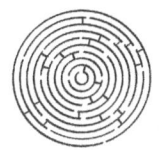

Day 34
A little more attention

Do a little more each day than you think you can.
- Lowell Thomas

Modern psychologists and ancient sages agree that our mind has a limited capacity for attention. It functions within a circle of attention. This means that the attention you give to selected items results in your mind being *less available* to notice other things. Where you focus your attention then becomes extremely important as focusing in certain directions can bring you satisfaction, happiness and peace of mind, whilst focusing in other directions causes unnecessary and avoidable pain and suffering. The good news is when you pay attention to your energy it enables you to connect to what really matters so you can show up *fully engaged*.

Do you remember the legendary detective Sherlock Holmes who developed an extraordinary sense of awareness and perceptiveness? Where others saw nothing unusual he noticed tiny but important clues, giving him a remarkable ability to read others and environments and thereby solve complex mysteries. The same quality of effectiveness can be developed with your energy, and it can prove just as valuable in helping you find clues to what makes your life successful for you. Such awareness includes you noticing details of ordinary behavior, other people's as well as your own. To become present in your life and to show up whole in your energy, it is not enough for you to be physically present, you need to bring your emotions, your mind and your divine connections out to play too, giving them a place of expression in your life.

Others notice when you pay attention, they like being around you as you validate their energy. In your life you have probably known at least a few people who felt like they truly listened and saw you, without being distracted by anyone or anything else. And you probably felt good around them as their *radiant energy* will have *recharged* yours. Unfortunately they are the unusual ones, so they stand out in a crowd. It's not because they listen, as most of us listen, but as we do so we allow ourselves to be continuously distracted by our own thoughts and feelings amongst other things. We filter another person's messages through our own filters of perception and as a result we are not quite there with each other.

My request then is that you *give a little bit more attention*, do a little more than you think you can. Be fully present with yourself and fully present with others in your life. Focus on learning to get as close as you can to understanding another person's reality as it is for them.

If you give a little more attention you will be rewarded with a whole lot more energy and a more rewarding life.

- *Simply breathe and relax into your meditation*
- *Light a candle and bring all of your attention to the candle*
- *Breathe deeply and evenly, allow your focus to shift entirely onto the candle*
- *Notice when you become distracted and without judgement bring yourself back to the candle*
- *Focus on keeping all of your attention with the candle*
- *Breathe openly and meditate on how you can develop this skill within your life*

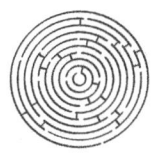

Day 35
Letting go

You have to give up the life you have
to get the life that is waiting for you.
- James Hillman

The pull into holding onto things is very strong. The exploration of our self is inextricably interwoven with the unfolding of our life. The natural ups and downs of life can either generate personal growth or create personal fears. It is where we feel fear that we usually also experience a *tightness* urging us to hold on. Once we also realize that most of us have a notion of learning as adding more fuel to the fire, acquiring *more* of something, be it skills or knowledge, we can just keep piling in the new stuff. Our internal mind can become like a dusty attic filled with junk and in desperate need of a clearing out.

In my role as a coach I have learned that most of us need to unlearn something before our mind can be open enough to embrace anything new. We need to let go of the years of clutter which keep us trapped in the same stuff, with the same beliefs and the same people year after year. Now don't get me wrong here there is nothing wrong with living your life from this place as long as you are 100% fulfilled doing so and for most of us that is not enough. *We feel called to more.*

If you truly want to grow spiritually, you'll realize that *keeping your stuff is what is keeping you trapped - you need to let go*. If you don't come to this place willingly I can guarantee your life will take you there kicking and screaming. I have seen this happen to myself and my clients so many times. Eventually you will want out, sometimes at any cost. Life will surround you with people and situations that will stimulate your growth, urging you to open your heart in the face of anything and everything and permit the letting go to take place. In truth your life has been doing this all along, it's just that now you realize the opportunity for you to let go of whatever is no longer serving you well in your life. Once clear, your energy is activated and magnetizes to you whatever you need to learn to let go. *So listen to your self.* You know what you need to release. Do it *while you still have a choice.* If you fail to let go and you hold on, chances are you will experience a sequence of events so quickly you won't know what hit you. You can find yourself *falling* instead.

Always let go as soon as you are aware that you didn't. Don't waste your time and energy holding on. Don't fall. Let go. *No matter what it is, let it go.* You are a great being who has been given a tremendous opportunity to explore beyond yourself. Let go of all your blockages and disturbances allowing them to *fuel* your journey. That which is holding you down can become a powerful force that raises you up. You merely have to be willing.

- *Breathe deeply and realize what it is within you that needs to be released. What is holding you back?*
- *Breathe in and know that you are separate from what needs to be released*
- *Go into your core and center yourself*
- *Let go and remain in your awareness. Don't allow any disturbed thoughts or feelings to knock you off your center*
- *Breathe out deeply and release. Just let it all go.*
- *Repeat as necessary*

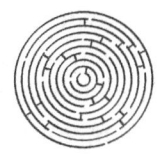

Day 36
Wounded heart

Have a heart that never hardens,
a temper that never tires
and a touch that never hurts.
- Charles Dickens

Live with an open heart. You cannot grow on a soul level if your heart remains closed. When your heart is open you stay receptive to yourself and others and channel positive emotions into your life by receiving and giving love freely. This can be challenging as our primal instincts direct us towards protection and in our civilized western world this has evolved from the physical protection of primitive societies into psychological protection. *We now experience the need to defend our self concepts rather than our bodies.* Our major struggles can end up being with our own inner fears, insecurities and destructive behavior patterns rather than with outside forces. Our challenge if we choose to accept it, is to transcend our heart's tendency to close.

You will come to a point in your development where you understand that if *you protect yourself you will never be free*. It's impossible. If you close and protect yourself, you are locking away this scared, insecure person within your heart. You can never be free that way. It keeps you small and limits your opportunities for growth. Your life can become stagnant and you become bored. If you really want to grow you have to do the opposite. Real spiritual growth happens when your heart is open and your energy is aligned. It happens when there is only one of you inside, not a part of you that's scared and a part of you that's not. You become unified within and as a consequence your energy becomes whole. From this place *your heart is willing to stay open*. Your heart has an energetic shield that you can use to engage whenever you are subject to extreme pain, anxiety or trauma but it is not intended to be in place permanently. If you erect such armor you cut off your energy from everything including yourself. An outpouring of love is the most potent healing vibration on Earth. If you have an open heart, every obstacle in your life eventually gives way because nothing in the world can resist this energy indefinitely. The more you love, the more energetically attractive you become and you begin to magnetize everything that you need directly to you.

Look around you, it is obvious when someone has closed their heart as their eyes are dull and their energy feels cold and dense. They have no warmth and lack the ability to truly connect with others. If you feel in danger of this happening to you, connect back to your energy with positive intention. *The spirit in you is greater than any injury you have ever experienced.* The most powerful way to recover this part of yourself is through self-love. Forgive yourself and others, release yourself from criticism and reconnect through prayer to your Higher Self. You may also benefit from movement, exercise and physical activity, anything to get your energy moving. Once you reconnect to your energy you can reclaim your right to live peacefully in your body, free from invasion by others and with a heart free to fully love again.

- *Breathe simply and fully*
- *Imagine your heart opening fully to yourself and to others within your life*
- *Consciously practice sending love and light to everyone you encounter, especially those who are difficult or injure your heart*
- *Be patient and affectionate in your appreciation of others. Be generous in your spirit.*
- *Laugh out loud and allow yourself to enjoy what brings you joy in every day*

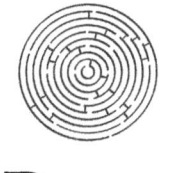

Day 37
Balanced energy

We are born to be directors of energy

Yes, there is such a thing! It is possible to be relatively balanced throughout your energy system without becoming an enlightened master! So what about you and your energy?

Balanced energy arises naturally when individuals have been actively involved in their own personal and spiritual growth. If you have balanced energy you will tend to be aware of your own physicality and have worked on your own healing, usually in energetic ways. You are likely to be a lifelong learner too, understanding that your own energetic system is *dynamic and constantly changing*. You are conscious that you need to enter into regular energetic practice to continuously attend to the needs of your energy ecosystem. You can cleanse and clear energy blockages as they arise.

A balanced energy system indicates a person who is well grounded, with a strong sense of body awareness and will be thriving in good health. They would be aware of their emotions without being ruled by them and would enjoy an active sexual life. The balanced third energy level would bring them self esteem and confidence without the need to control or dominate others. They would be centered and peaceful with an open and loving heart. Others would gravitate towards them since they are likely to have a strong sense of presence. They actively listen to others yet are also able to express their own ideas with truth and clarity. The higher energy levels would also bring them imagination, wisdom and a personal connection with spirit. Sounds good?

Since our energy is dynamic and constantly changing, in many ways a balanced energy system is an ideal which we can all work towards. By using your strengths to support your weaker energy levels, and by treating yourself with loving kindness, you too have the potential to achieve balance. As you learn more about your energy you will intuitively know when things are out of sync. As with all new skills, it becomes only a matter of time, patience and commitment to your individual energy practice.

- *As you move through your day today, ask yourself what would bring balance to your life?*
- *Explore what would bring balance to your energy*
- *What do you need to attend to physically? emotionally? mentally? spiritually?*
- *How committed are you to achieving balance? What difference would that make?*
- *Breathe and commit to doing what needs to be done*

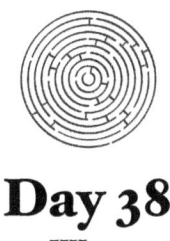

Day 38
Water

Like water, be gentle and strong.
Gentle enough to follow the natural curves and
wonders of the earth and
strong enough to rise up and reshape the world.
- Brenda Peterson

I love water, it re-energizes me in a way that no other element of nature can. I love the water for its fluidity, its softness and ability to fill whatever hole it finds. It has the power to flow into life embracing anything which covers its path, and over time it shapes our world with its quiet transformations.

It seems to me that we all should embrace love like water. We seem to waste much of our energy wondering who is worthy of our love when at the deepest elemental sense, this is not really our choice. We don't choose this out pouring of emotion anymore than the river chooses where to flow. Without our interference our love would embrace everyone, knowing at an intimate level that *we don't ever run out of love* we always have more than enough to give. In truth the more we let love flow through our lives, the more we have to love. It is beneath the many choices that we make in our lives that it is the essence of love, just like the water, that flows back into the world through us.

Love like water then, is about extending your love and letting it wash over the life in and around you. It means for you to extend your love, concern and caring towards everyone and everything you meet, including animals, places and our environment. It is about going beyond our usual definitions of love and expanding our consciousness to understand how we can play our part on the planet in contribution, community and service. This is not about grand gestures but small well placed intentions. It is about moving into action in your local community and playing your part. You can express your love for others by volunteering your services in your community, being an energy conscious consumer or recycling resources to help others. *It is about doing what you can while you can, nothing more and nothing less.*

Think of your love like the water, an endless stream of positive energy flowing out from your heart; gentle enough to embrace everything in its path and yet with a quiet strength that has the cumulative power to really make a difference, in not only your world, but the world in which we all live.

- *Go and find some water and sit in front of it*
- *Notice the flow of movement, the quiet gentle power of the water*
- *Feel the energy within the water and feel the energy within you*
- *Feel your energy flow like water, from within out into the world*
- *Imagine your vibration rising steadily as you embrace others with your energy*
- *Imagine embracing the whole world*
- *As you go about your day today imagine yourself fluid and flowing like the water, embracing all that comes your way*

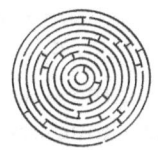

Day 39
The risk to bloom

And the time came when the risk
to remain tight in a bud was more painful
than the risk it took to blossom.
- Anais Nin

We all face this turning point many times in the cycle of our lives, when resisting the flow of inner events suddenly feels more hurtful than doing the thing that we fear most - leaping into the unknown. There is no way of knowing for sure when is the best time to shift ourselves, no-one else can help us with our struggle. It is something only we can know for ourself, by *listening* and *responding* to the well of our emotions.

How often do we get in our own way? We give ourselves numerous reasons why now is not the right time. Our need to stay in our comfort zone, to cling to the familiar compels us to hold on tightly to our lives, often squeezing out the last sign of life. *How bad do things need to get before we realize it would be less painful to face our fears?* I have friend who owns a beautiful flower shop, and she tells me that roses that won't open are nicknamed bullets. They are thrown away because they will never bloom. They have turned inwards on themselves to such an extent that they can never release their petals or their fragrance. I have certainly known a few people who can relate to the problem of the roses.

As a coach it always fascinates and somehow humbles me, when I realize again how the risk to bloom can seem so insurmountable beforehand and so liberating once the decision to bloom has been made and the threshold has been crossed. It reminds me of a very dear client who I have worked with now for many years. Upon meeting her for the first time, she found herself unable to articulate her challenges instead showing me with her hands which she curled up really tightly, until her knuckles were white. In tears she symbolically showed me that what she wanted to do was to unfurl her hands but it was so frightening to her she had *no idea* how or even where to begin. It was a revelation for her to realize that the pain of staying tightly shut was more painful than the risk it took to open. With gentle coaxing she slowly unravelled and found that her fears were not realized.

This is the same for most of us, our fears are usually far greater than we experience in reality when we eventually step out regardless. The same can be said of me during my worst health challenges. There came a time when the pain of remaining severely incapacitated, giving up all hope of recovery became greater than my fear of holding out the hope that I could somehow heal myself. Either path seemed painful so it became something of a non decision. My survival instinct kicked in and intuitively I followed. We can all flower in an instant, as soon as the pain of not flowering and not loving ourselves enough to change, becomes greater than our fears.

- *Find a quiet space and identify what scares you most about being truly who you are in the world*
- *As you meditate imagine your guardian angels, looking over you in protection, encouraging you to step out in the direction of your fears*
- *Feel into your center, ground yourself and sense what it feels like to open your vulnerability, if even for a moment*
- *Without telling anyone, choose a point in your day today to open yourself just a little more to life*
- *Repeat this whenever you feel yourself contracting and you start to feel your sense of things tighten*

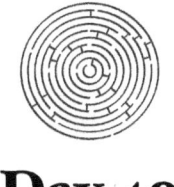

Day 40
Flow of love

I think one must finally take one's life in one's arms.
- Arthur Miller

The foundation of all of our loving emerges from our ability to love ourselves. We can only love another to the extent to which we have learned to love ourselves. It is the force which pervades all of our thoughts and actions and seeks to expand or inhibit the flow of our love in any given moment. *The simple truth is that in loving ourselves we love the world.* Yet how do we do this without appearing self-centered and arrogant?

There is no doubt that it can be challenging at times, a little like trying to bite your own teeth as your life crashes on unexplained shores and you do your best to reclaim what parts of yourself have survived. *Love requires courage, and loving yourself requires a courage unlike any other.* It needs us to stay loyal to ourselves, to continue to believe in our own sense of self-worth, our capabilities and the inner truth, which no-one else can see or experience in quite the same way. No-one else has the same level of V.I.P. access that we do to our internal machinations and so no-one else can validate our opinion of self. We must find our own sense of security and we must *nurture* our inner relationship. Until we begin to love ourselves fully, embracing ourselves wholly with all of our being we struggle to give and receive within the flow of love.

During my darkest days of my pain, I recall being confronted with myself. I longed for a day without pain and like a child who doesn't want to play anymore I found myself wondering about the "off" switch for life. It was then that I felt myself rise from within, did I not care for myself enough to continue? Where was the love? Was I really going to accept the views of strangers who said I would ever recover or did I love myself enough to take a different path? The realization hit me right between the eyes, I didn't love myself, in fact my inner self hated my physical body. I blamed my body for letting me down, for causing me pain, for taking away my life. The emotions were so overwhelming I had no choice but to let them through (they were coming anyway) the inner rage was deafening until black and blue I retreated. I was done. Exhausted. Collapsed. It was at that point I felt an overwhelming surge of love for myself, a sadness for everything I was going through and a great compassion for my body. It was my time to embrace myself and begin to build a new relationship with myself, physically, emotionally, mentally and spiritually. I had *reconnected to my light* and was allowing it to define what became a positive and energetic foundation for my healing.

When we embrace the light within and we believe what no-one else can see, it is here that we find we are each other. We are ultimately connected in all moments of living. We can find that in our very core, *at the very center of our self we find the world and we are one.* It is here where the energy flows and the light floods in. It is here where we return to the very core of our loving; our ability to give and receive.

- *Breathe deeply and return to your core*
- *Close your eyes and turn your attention to your heart center*
- *Feel your heart beating carrying with it waves of love energy*
- *With each breath feel into your experience of love, allowing it to expand in your consciousness*
- *Imagine yourself stood directly in front of you - notice your energy physically, emotionally, mentally and spiritually - notice the wounds, the fears and anxieties around yourself and love. Be compassionate with yourself.*
- *Open your arms and embrace yourself fully. Love*

Recorded by the author, **'An Energetic Journey'** is a free Guided Meditation that accompanies this book.

For your copy, go to: **https://rebrand.ly/AEA-Meditation**

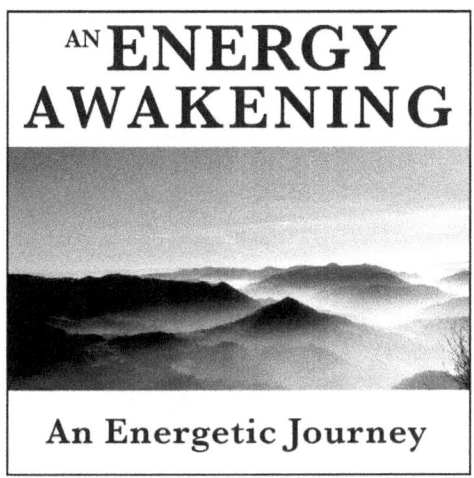

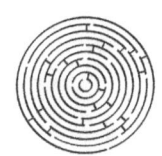

Part Three: Finding Freedom

I know but one freedom and that is the freedom of the mind.

- Antoine De Saint Expuery

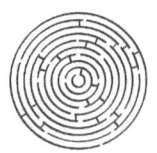

Day 41
Getting real

Go beyond the impersonation, beyond boundaries and limitations.
Insist on yourself.

Do yourself a favor, be *authentic* and be *real*. Everyone knows when you are not. One of the biggest problems we encounter when communicating with each other is that we often forget that *our communication has multiple energetic levels*. When these are not aligned in the speaker, the listener will receive mixed signals and will become confused. Conversely, when these levels are aligned communication is smooth, authentic and in flow.

Behind your words your energy is communicating an invisible stream of your emotions, motivations, goals and intentions so it pays to learn more about yourself so you can ensure that your communication is authentic and in line with your sense of self and well-being.

As the Earth keeps turning and night becomes day, we have no choice but to turn towards what we feel is real; anything else merely *drains our energy*. It is an interesting challenge and one I have struggled with my entire life. Like most of us when I am faced with overwhelming challenges in my life, my survival instincts compel me to hold back what feels real. When someone says something that hurts me or circumstances in my life take a downturn I have learned to absorb the impact and pretend that nothing has changed. I am a master at putting a smile on my face, holding my head high and continuing with my life as though everything is fine. This was a particular challenge for me when suffering with my health, it took over a year of struggle before I faced my overwhelming pain and admitted even to myself that I was really ill. It was as though by pretending to myself that everything was fine I would never actually become ill. Wrong. I was a classic case of denial and worse still I was really good at it. When I eventually gave in and retreated to lick my wounds most people were startled and had no idea of what I was putting myself through. My energy, however, was exhausted just when I needed it most.

It is simple and yet so brave for us to admit that we are hurt when we are hurt, scared when we are scared and sad when we are sad. In many situations in every single day I notice how this desire for authenticity, this energy of realness challenges me. It calls me forth *to live life naked and from my truth*. When I do, I notice how this expression of what is real for me releases a strong vibrant energy that influences my life and those around me. It enables me to shine my light out into the Universe and I notice how it calls forth others to come out from behind themselves, belly up in their vulnerability and participate in the realness of the moment.

- *Center yourself and begin to breathe deeply*
- *Let your thoughts begin to rise within you and come into your conscious awareness*
- *Notice what is raw and real for you right now*
- *Be careful to voice your feelings as yours. Using I statements "I feel..."*
- *Lean into your sense of real*
- *During your day listen to yourself like never before. Be mindful of how the pulse of what is real for you shifts around. Notice what you do with it. Notice when you are able to be real*
- *Each day choose one moment to come into your life and be truly, authentically real. Notice what happens to your energy*

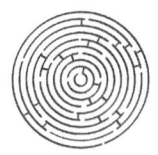

Day 42
Passion

The point of passion is mainly to follow,
to let yourself love what you love,
to respect your hunger and obey your thirst.
- Greg Levoy

Each of us is called to become a person unique in all time. You have a legacy designed specifically for you. No-one else can feel your passion or bring forth your signature presence. Your passion will differ from others because it comes *through* you, filtered through your life experiences, your values, ethics, family, cultural background and beliefs. *Connecting to your passion is really about saying yes to your inner calling.* It is about finding and doing what you love to do. If you simply do what you love, you will always love what you do and that sounds like a recipe for a successful and well-lived life to me.

It sounds so simple and yet many people struggle with this simple notion and settle for less, *much less*. They may even end up living someone else's life, always aiming to please everyone else and forgetting themselves. Don't let this be you. Aim to explore your own brilliance and the magnificence of your own voice, your essence and your passion. *Listen to your soul's calling.*

When you recognize, accept and respond to your life's calling you can live with passionate intention and direction. Others will notice and respond. When you say *"yes"* to your dreams and connect them together with your passion, you can reach your highest potential. If you are unsure of your calling, then listen to your uncertainty. Be patient with yourself. I have learned over the years that responding to a calling is not merely a one time deal but a lifelong process, always in motion, always evolving. Your responses are likely to be a meandering process rather than a straight line. *Move forward at a pace that is right for you.* Float around for a while as this may open you to somewhere different than you expected. Your calling will find you, but will you find it? Trust your feelings, if it feels right, it usually is.

Life is so much better when your passion and calling, fall into step together and become aligned. Know what you love to do and do more of it. Be passionate, nothing boosts your personal energy faster.

- *Find some space to go into your energy and connect to your passion*
- *Feel it rise within your body, filling you with positive sensations*
- *Breathe into your passion, let it rise out of you and into the light*
- *Let your passion expand your heart*
- *Breathe deeply and get ready to follow your passion in today and tomorrow*

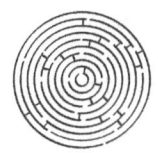

Day 43
No need for approval

Do just once what others say you can't do,
and you will never pay attention
to their limitations again.
- James R Cook

Let me tell you a secret that will change your life. This is *your* life designed especially for *you* to live it how *you* choose. No excuses. *You always have a choice.* Nobody else can define your life for you, it always comes down to your decision about how you live it. It is your opportunity to establish your unique expression in the world - and if you don't live your life who will?

Taking time to consider what is truly important in your life, and relaxing your grip on what is not, can enable the simple truths for living a meaningful life more visible to you. You can detach from the physical world, from others and things. By all means be part of the daily activity of life just don't be *enslaved* by it. You can live a fully integrated life becoming a vibrant part of your community, having fun with family and friends, just don't depend on anything outside of your spirit to make you feel happy. Your inner peace does not come from anything outside of you; not the acquisition of material things, the attainment of fulfilling relationships or the approval of others. These bring only short term gains and the danger is that you open yourself up to far more disappointment when your sense of self depends upon others for you to feel okay. You cannot make the Universe around you or the people in it *do, feel or think* what you want, no matter how much you may believe that you can persuade others, or even how hard you may try.

Freeing your soul is not easy since we are all attached to someone or something. Our worldly attachments and our affections for people we love enrich our lives. And it isn't merely people and things we are attached to either, we can be attached to our usual ways of thinking, our self-images, the habit of conforming to the customs of those around us and ideas about how we are supposed to act. *We can even become attached to being not attached to everyone and everything!* Although the idea of non attachment would be very liberating in some ways, as a busy mom of three it also seems a little extreme. I wonder if we can ever truly let what we have been attached to float away without fighting the emotional tides of a sense of loss? *The truth is our attachments tug at our heartstrings.* Rightly or wrongly, I don't want to let go of the attachment to my children, but I can loosen my grip. The key for me has been to find those questionable attachments, those things that were not supportive of the way I wanted to live my life. As a consequence, I have found great value in developing a healthy respect for simplicity. It is this which has enabled me to avoid the troubles I can get into when I become entangled as a result of my attachments.

A turning point is when you realize that your desire for approval from others is not likely to be something you will get all of the time, from all of the people. They have different priorities, so don't depend on it, as this is a thankless task that can only lead to unhappiness. Let go of others' expectations and *live your life your way*, at least then there will be one person who will be pleased with the outcome.

- *This is an awareness exercise. As you go through your day today, stay present and aware.*
- *Notice whether you are complying with how others want you to be. How do the views of others affect you? Are you seeking approval?*
- *Are you living from your truth or withholding who you really are?*
- *After each interaction, take a deep breath and return to the fullness of who you are*

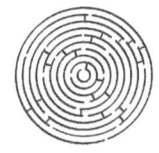

Day 44
The lost art of wanting

What is it that YOU want?

Many of us have trouble wanting for ourselves. This is not surprising as many of us grew up with models of behavior which frowned upon wanting as being selfish and unspiritual. This is a terrible shame as wanting is *really good* on many different levels. It may also be the one essential ingredient needed to follow your inner voice and become truly who you are. *Only wanting has the energy or even the power to bring about transformational change.* Wanting is the motivation of the Universe acting within you, gathering momentum and expanding Creation.

Your true wants are a the very core of your soul, they express your individuality and are as unique and individual as your fingerprints. It is what you choose to do with your wants that defines you and the quality of your life. I have met many clients who take convoluted paths to ignore or avoid them, expending large amounts of energy to deny their very existence. Some sneak around in denial. They hide behind themselves to avoid them and this can become a habit, developing unhindered into becoming the story of their lives. Wanting can be the very thing that decides whether your life was happy or sad for you.

One thing is for sure, no matter what anyone tells you, trying to avoid your wants or even compromise them doesn't get rid of them, not even for a moment. And it does drain your energy making life a lot less fun. *So what is it that you truly want?* If you allow yourself to really consider this, it can be very difficult. Even after you get past your concerns about being selfish, almost inevitably you will start to wonder how impossible it would be for you, as you worry about whether you are wasting your time on an idle pipe dream. It can be easier to only allow "safe" wants through our filters as anything more could represent the ability to derail your entire life! There's nothing wrong with the safer wants except they only express a very small measure of your true wanting. There is no harm in knowing. After all, what you do with your knowing is up to you.

Dare to open the gateway to your deepest desires and ask yourself what would get you truly excited? What would really increase your life energy? What would give you the maximum amount of pleasure and joy? What wold be 100% for you? Now sit back and really listen to your answers...

- *Be still with yourself and listen to your responses to the above questions*
- *Meditate deeply on the question - what is it that I truly want?*
- *Be ready to be raw with yourself, open yourself to a different level of possibility. Learn what lies unhindered within your very soul*
- *Listen to your heart's deepest desires and develop a true sense of knowing what it is you truly want*

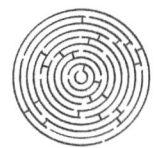

Day 45
Your infinite energy

You have a wellspring of beautiful energy inside of you.
When you are open you feel it;
when you are closed you don't.
- M. Singer

Consciousness is one of the great mysteries in life, energy is another. It is actually a real shame how little attention we pay to energy in the West, especially our inner energy. We study the energy outside and give great value to our energy resources, but we have somehow managed to ignore the energy within. *Most people go about their lives on a daily basis without really understanding what is going on in their energetic system.* They fail to realize that every thought, every action, every emotion is an expenditure of energy. Absolutely everything in our lives requires an investment of energy. *Where does all this energy come from?*

We all have an inner source of energy and the ability to make huge shifts in our energy at a moments notice. If you doubt this, think about a time in your life when you were so worried about something it depressed your energy, e.g. finances; you had no money and were feeling down and drained. Nothing seemed to help and you had little or no energy. Next you receive a telephone call to say you have won over a million dollars on the lottery. For months and months you had no energy and then in a matter of seconds there is so much energy it blows you away. This flow of energy comes from the very depths of your being. You should all know about this energy because it is *yours.* It belongs to you as your birthright and its unlimited. You can harness it any time you want. It has nothing to do with the food you eat or the shape you are in physically. It doesn't depend on age and it never gets tired. This is your spiritual energy and all it needs from you to flow effortlessly in your life is your *openness* and *receptivity*.

You have the ability to close down your energy and block its flow. When you close, your energy stops flowing. When you open all the energy rushes up inside of you and is available to support you in your life. *You* have control, you can decide how much of this energy you would like access to and then commit to staying open to it. You stay open by never closing. It really is a simple as that. Closing is a habit, and like any other habit it can be broken. You should never leave anything as important as your energy flow to chance. If you want more energy, and most of us do then don't ever close. The more you can teach yourself to stay open, the more energy can flow into you. Any time you feel yourself starting to close ask yourself whether it really is in your best interests to cut off your energy flow. You can learn to stay open no matter what happens to you in your life. *You simply decide not to close.*

The most important thing in your life is your energy, without it you literally can't do anything. If you are always tired, then life is no fun. But if you're always inspired and full of vitality then every minute of every day is an exciting experience. If you love life, (and I hope you do!) nothing is ever worth closing over.

- *Breathe deeply and begin to drop inside of yourself to check in with your energy*
- *Give your energy your full attention - is it open or closed?*
- *Allow it to open just a little more than usual. Allow your energy to enter you and take it with you throughout your day*
- *Every time you feel the urge to close your energy today, take a deep breath and allow yourself to remain a little more open than last time*

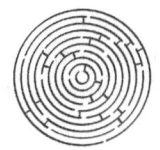

Day 46
Stop the world

There is no such thing as bad weather, only the wrong clothes

Once whilst I was on retreat in the Lake District, England on a cold winter's day my meditation teacher came to my side and asked me "*How is the world treating you?*" I mumbled some general response that things were okay and then she asked me "*And how are you treating the world?*" I was a little shocked as I had never thought about it in that way before. In fact if I was being honest with myself, it was my belief that I had managed to stop the world. I had "got off" for a short time, leaving the world behind somewhat by going on this retreat. As I let her comments sink in, and reflected upon them I realized that there is no leaving the world, that even on retreat I was somehow relating to the world in every breath and in every moment. I knew then, as I still do today that I have a lot to learn about why I am here (or even there) in the first place, what meditation is all about for me and *underlying everything the stunning question of what was I really doing with my life?*

Ever since that time those two questions have never really left me as I now understand that we are in an intimate relationship with the world in every moment. It is a relationship which defines and shapes our lives. It is a dance of continual give and take, of how our internal relates to the external, and yet it is very easy to become sucked into the illusion that those two questions are separate, between out there and in here. I know at a deep level our external world is usually a mirror image of what is going on internally for us. It is how our energy relates to the field.

There have been many times when I have noticed myself wanting to force things to be a certain way, to do things "my way", to push against the flow of life and in hindsight I notice how that merely isolates me from my possibilities. This is where I cut myself off from my energy flow by refusing to acknowledge how things actually are, usually because they are not how I want them to be. *Do you know what I mean?*

I slowly learned that I could stop imposing my will on my life and start to live my truth. I could get out of my own way (and everybody else's). I had the opportunity to enter into my own life stream and allow interesting new possibilities to emerge. I had to stop my old world from spinning before I could enter the new.

As each new day dawns I have a choice of what to do with the time I have been given and for that I am particularly grateful. As do you. You can *choose* how to spend your days and really begin to live your life, whilst you have what in the big scheme of human evolution is merely a short time to live.

- *Close your eyes and consider your relationship to the world*
- *Meditate on those two questions : "How is the world treating you?" and "How are you treating the world?"*
- *What do you notice?*
- *Breathe into your thoughts and then release them into the day*
- *Go out into your day and treat the world the way you would like to be treated back*
- *Smile!*

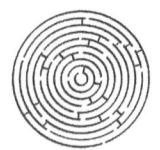

Day 47
Moment to moment

Wherever we go, wherever we are,
whatever is happening and no matter what time it is
or what the calendar says,
we always have only moments to live.
- Jon Kabbat-Zinn

Are you ready for the adventure of your lifetime? Are you ready to step into your life in a mindful way, to become present in every moment, to be awake in the here and now? The first step on this adventure is to cultivate a particular kind of awareness known as mindfulness. This is what essentially makes us human. Mindfulness is cultivated by paying attention to the *moments* in our lives and ultimately realizing that it is *only in the moments that we can ever truly live.*

It does demand that you pay attention to your life *as though it really mattered, as though you really mattered*. It requires that you be motivated to understand *who you really are* at a deeper level in any given moment and be aware of *who you are becoming*. As dynamic as life is, we soon realize that who we once were is not actually who we are today, in fact we can change considerably from moment to moment. This is where we need to dig beyond the surface traits and behaviors to reclaim the essence within. It involves cultivating all of our senses, reclaiming our energy and observing ourselves when we feel deeply insecure. It demands we catch ourselves as we try to use all of our resources to control as tightly as possible, all the variables in our external world, usually an impossible and exhausting activity as we learn that striving is often counter-productive.

Consider this your wake-up call to mobilize your powerful inner resources to use your energy for healing, and radiating a positive energy out into the world. You have more senses than you think. In addition to your knowing, what you are seeing, hearing, tasting, smelling and touching; you also have your conscious thought, your mind and your intuition. Then there is proprioception (the body knowing how it is positioned in space) and interoception (the overall feel of the body as a whole). Once you can establish a relationship with all of your senses you will begin to connect with the more subtle energies of the higher levels and become more intensely alive.

- *Find some space and stop yourself, intentionally waking up to how things are in this very moment*
- *Sit down and allow yourself to drop into presence, drop into the moment*
- *Be still with yourself*
- *Go behind all of your thinking, behind your knowing, behind the doing and see what is there*
- *Notice what is*
- *Lean into your moments, open a little more to your moments and live your life a little larger*

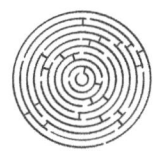

Day 48
Playing small

Make no small plans for they have no power to stir the soul.
- Niccolo Machiavelli

Recently I read about an experiment where a scientist raised some baby fish in a small glass tank, which was inside of a larger tank that held adult fish. The baby fish in the smaller tank could see the adult fish in the larger tank, but because of the glass barrier they couldn't swim out. Once the small fish had grown, the researcher removed the glass walls of the small tank so they could swim out, but they didn't. They stayed in exactly the same place that used to be contained within their walls. The habit and memory of their small world was more real to them than the freedom that was possible now that the glass had been removed. They never explored their edges. They played *small*.

Like these fish, many of us have become accustomed to our own limited environment believing that this smaller, safer place is the only way we can survive. We may be aware of the edges of our comfort zone and yet fool ourselves into believing that we can fulfill our potential by accepting the environment we have been given, even when it doesn't fit us that well. *Our quality of life and the quality of our energy is not served by us playing small.* Our passion grows dim and our ability to fulfill our purpose and find our wisdom remains hidden. We hide our light for fear of risking the stability of which we have grown accustomed.

You can give yourself much more space to expand by asking yourself what is it that would bring out the *best* in you. What are the living conditions that *empower* you instead of *imprisoning* you? What are the elements that you need to have in your life so that you can grow an authentic and generous life?

You are a living ecosystem of energy and as such, you have a unique environment in which you particularly will flourish. It is your challenge to define that for yourself. As humans we all have an innate need to be constantly growing and learning. Your energy also needs to be moving in a rhythm that allows your mind, body, soul and heart to be in alignment. This can be difficult to achieve when you are feeling constrained. The smaller the space within which you live the less opportunity there is for a free flow of energy and movement. When you play small you not only do yourself a disservice but also everyone else out there in the world who is waiting patiently for you share your gifts. Those people whose lives will be positively affected by your energy being out in the world.

Have no doubt, it is our purpose as humans to evolve. Evolution demands that we continuously stretch ourselves beyond our limitations, it encourages us to expand and play a bigger game. No more playing small, it dims your light and doesn't allow you to shine!

- *Sit quietly and bring to mind your plans for the future*
- *How can you play a bigger game?*
- *What is one change you are afraid to make in your life, that if you succeeded would give you a more expansive environment in which to grow?*
- *Breathe deeply and ask yourself what are you waiting for?*
- *Breathe gently and empty your mind. Don't worry now about what to do, exhale and feel the wisdom to evolve waiting inside of you*

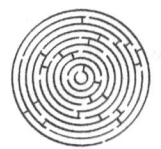

Day 49
Open your mind

Minds are like parachutes, they only function when open.
- Thomas Dewar

Think for yourself. Yes, I know it sounds obvious but in my experience it really isn't. *Over 80% of all the issues people carry around in their personal energy systems are given to them by someone else.* From a young age we are taught what it means to be compliant and please other people and somewhere along the *way we get lost in our own lives.* Get to know yourself, your beliefs, opinions and identity. Separate out what is *your* thinking and what belongs to someone else. Form some opinions, know your own values and be clear on what it is you stand for. You know what they say, if you don't stand for something you will fall for anything! Consider if your thinking is working for you in your life, if not discard it and think something else. You don't have to choose to be and do today, who you were and what you did yesterday. You can open your mind to a new and more exciting possibility.

You may have heard me talk about the two groups of people you can choose to be around in your life; the radiators and the drains. If you want to be successful in life as in business you need to look after yourself and your energy, so it pays to spend time around those who energize you and lift you up with their energy and enthusiasm. *Hang out with big thinkers and positive people.* These are the people who can urge you to think bigger than you would naturally do by yourself and help you to believe you can play a bigger game. Go spend a few hours with them and notice how your mind opens to more expansive possibilities and how great you feel just to be alive.

When you open your mind, leaving your comfort zone can become a way of life, so you may as well get used to it! There's a great saying that I have stuck on my office noticeboard it says "*Do something that scares you every day!*". Why not? If you want to live a life worth living you need to find the courage to step outside of yourself and be challenged, be frightened and be stimulated. You need to come out from behind yourself and get real. If you don't, you run the risk of becoming boring and stagnant. Your relationships will suffer and others will pass you by without a backward glance.

Expanding your comfort zone, like expanding your mind makes you feel good about yourself. It makes you feel alive and gives you extra confidence. Life is a learning journey, we are continuously adapting and growing and you will never know the extent of your own potential unless you give yourself a chance. In the words of Susan Jeffers :"Feel the fear and do it anyway!"

- *Find some space and begin to breathe deeply*
- *Close your eyes and feel into the space beneath your feet, feel into the floor which support you, the ground underneath you stretching deep down into the earth*
- *Now feel into the air above your head, that stretches up into the clouds and further into the Universe, going into infinity*
- *Open your mind a little further to embrace a larger more expansive perspective of you*
- *Notice how it feels to open your mind, allow your thoughts to come streaming in. Listen*
- *Breathe deeply and know your mind is yours to open whenever you choose*

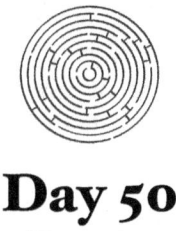

Day 50
Knowing

Even when I can't remember,
a deeper part of me always knows.

Your sense of knowing is a gift which travels with you wherever you go. It is instinctive, primal, always bubbling away just below the surface. Even when you think you don't know, you usually do, but your *not knowing* is merely a protective mechanism shielding you from that which you are not ready or willing to know just yet.

If I were to ask you right now, what is it that you know to be true for you? What would you say? What is it that you know with certainty right now in this moment?

One of the easiest ways to get in touch with your sense of knowing is to get out of your head and drop into your body. Your body never lies. *When you can learn to read the messages of your body there is literally nothing you will not know.* Your body can tell you when you feel good about a certain person, or whether you are about to make a bad decision. It can tell you when it is time to rest or time to get your Mojo on. Your body is a sensitive instrument, a highway to your inner knowing which will tell you unfailingly what you are feeling at any given moment. It will always be telling you something, the real question is not whether you think you know something or not, *the real question is are you listening?*

One thing I know is that you are not in charge. You may think you are and I guess a few of you are wanting to argue with me right now, but control is an illusion. No matter how much time and energy you invest trying to control everything and everyone around you, it will never happen. Life has a way of showing you a different way as stuff happens, good and bad. I realize it may come as a shock to some of you, but you are not in charge of this world! No matter how much you want to be, no matter how much you want to control everything, no matter how much you think you are or deserve to be, you are NOT. And if you are not in charge then no-one else is either!

Once you accept this you can let go of so much stuff it really is *liberating*. You still have obligations, you need to be respectful of the world you live in and the people you live in it with. It's just that you don't have overall responsibility for running the whole show and everything in it. You can resign your position as Master of the Universe and open up some space to take yourself lightly. You are not now as busy as you may have thought. You get the opportunity to *laugh a little more and think a little less*. This is so important to remember and so easy to forget. Business and life don't have to be as serious as some people like to make out. Laughing at yourself and your situation has a double positive effect. Firstly it diffuses tension and helps you to regain a sense of proportion and secondly it has a real positive impact on your physical, emotional and mental energy. *It gives you an energy boost*. Laughter actually causes the release of endorphins which make you feel better as well as giving you a lighter perspective on life. Let your knowing be light and flow into the joyful stream of your life.

- *Center yourself and reconnect to the reality of your knowing*
- *Get out of your head and drop inside your body*
- *Let your breath take you, for the moment, beneath the surface into the depths of your knowing*
- *What do you know to be true?*
- *As you exhale, feel the expansiveness around all that you know*
- *As you inhale, deep within your core, feel the mystery where nothing is lacking*
- *Allow a small chunk of laughter to bubble up to the surface - smile, giggle, laugh. Release*

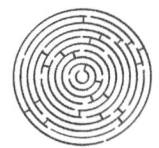

Day 51
A blossoming heart

The people that are the hardest to love
are usually the ones who need it the most.

The vocabulary of the heart covers a wide spectrum of emotion and experience, yet a blossoming heart depends on one of three contexts, all of which are relational; *self-love, love for others and divine love.* Needless to say the first blossoming of love is in relation to yourself. It means loving yourself with the same intensity that we typically reserve for others. You demonstrate self-love when you say *yes* to yourself and no to someone else's agenda, so that you can stay on track with your calling. Self-love is when you fully accept yourself regardless of your past, your behaviors or who you think yourself to be. It is the very foundation from which you can begin to love others. *The reality is that you cannot love anyone else fully until you are able to open your heart to yourself.*

Love for others is about relating in service, consciously serving as a steward for others. It is a rare person who is totally clear and comfortable with their own sense of self all of the time and it is rarer still to find someone who naturally empowers people wherever they go. If this is not you yet, don't worry! Most of us aren't but it is important that you acknowledge your power to influence others wherever you go. In all interactions we have the opportunity to love others, form connections and build relationships; we also have the power to give others positive feedback to make them feel good about themselves, (the opposite, is of course, also true). Why not give everyone you meet the gift of positive energy, notice the positive and share it with them? You will be radiating out from your blossoming heart and empowering yourself as well as everyone else you meet.

Divine love is the quality of love that extends beyond the cognitive, emotional and physical realms into the mystery of the Universe and the subtle energies that lie within. Divine love is experiencing a profound vision, appreciating a breathtaking view from the top of a mountain and discovering the intensity within a piece of art. Such experiences of awe and wonder are nourishing to your soul. You can also express your deep affinity with the Divine by honoring your true self, becoming real and authentic in everything you do.

We all wear the cloak of possibility. At its very core a blossoming heart is open to finding the passion within, about falling in love with your future so that you can devote your physical, emotional, mental and spiritual energy to be of service to yourself and others.

- *Find yourself a mirror and affirm your blossoming heart*
- *"I care about my own well-being and that of others, regardless of whether I know them personally"*
- *"I am following my passion and my calling, doing what I love and loving what I do"*
- *"I freely share my joy with others"*
- *Breathe deeply, find some space and notice what is coming up for you*
- *Breathe through any emotions*
- *Place your attention on your heart and feel it blossoming in your life*
- *As you go through your day today, notice the presence of your blossoming heart as it touches everyone you meet*

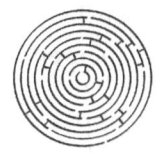

Day 52
Leaning into flow

Tomorrows fresh opportunities can't make their way
in a world full of yesterday's assumptions.

Flow is body and mind working together. It adds up to a sense of mastery or even better a sense of participation in the content of one's own life. Genuinely happy individuals are few and far between. How many people do you know who are 100% happy with what they are doing? Who are reasonably satisfied with their lot, who don't regret the past and look to the future with genuine confidence? You may know some, but I can guarantee it won;t be the majority. This says to me that there are not many people out there who are aware of and know how to work with their own energy to move themselves into flow. *But you are different! You can lean into flow.*

Flow happens when all of a persons relevant skills are needed to cope with the challenges of a situation and that person's attention is completely absorbed by the activity. There is no excess psychic energy left over to process any information but what the activity offers, as all the information is concentrated on the relevant stimuli. As a result people become so involved in what they are doing that the activity becomes spontaneous, almost automatic and they stop becoming aware of themselves as separate from the actions they are performing. It is this *total absorption* in an activity that people often describe as "flow". As one workshop participant explained about playing basketball "My concentration is complete. I become so involved in what I am doing that I am not aware of anything else, time seems to melt away - I just become totally involved in the game and sort of lose touch with the rest of the world. My energy runs really smoothly. I feel relaxed, comfortable and energetic. I'm in the zone."

Although the flow experience appears to be effortless it is far from being so, as it does not seem to happen without *some level of skilled performance* and any lapse in concentration will erase it. To live your life in flow provides a serious challenge as in daily life we keep interrupting what we do with questions and doubts. We often question the necessity of our actions and become judgmental or critical about the reasons why we are carrying them out. As we have seen in flow, there is no need for this level of reflection. This reflection just serves to *interrupt the flow*, the action itself is enough to carry us forward. What enables us to stay in flow is clear and immediate feedback and working towards clear goals.

Flow is intrinsically linked to improving the quality of your life. As any of you will know who have ever searched for a recipe for success or happiness - it doesn't exist - because optimal experience depends on the ability to control what happens in consciousness moment by moment and each person has to achieve this on the basis of their own individual efforts and creativity.

Control over your intuitive energy is not purely a cognitive skill. It requires the commitment of continued practice, of being present and noticing in the moment the messages from intuition, the physical body and the emotions. It is not enough to have read this book and know how to do it. You must practice consistently. Just as an athlete in flow has consistently practiced what they need to lean into their flow.

- *Center yourself and bring to mind the last time you felt in the flow*
- *Breathe fully and feel the intensity of the experience with your whole body*
- *Lean deeper into the experience*
- *What were you doing at the time?*
- *How can you experience more flow in your life?*
- *Lean in and allow*

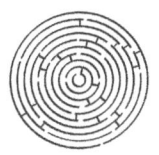

Day 53
Forgiveness

The weak can never forgive.
Forgiveness is the attribute of the strong.
- Gandhi

One of the most difficult things about healing after we have been hurt by others, is how to put those wounds to rest when those who have hurt us will not admit to their part in causing the pain. We often think about forgiveness as external to ourselves, that we forgive other people for them. When in reality *forgiving others is simultaneously an act of kindness towards yourself,* as it can sometimes serve to heal your painful memories. As resentments grow in your emotional energy they become like a cloud filming the clarity of your energy. There may seem to be a million good reasons to hang onto them but I can guarantee they are just a million ways to drain your energy. You might even get an energetic charge from all that resentment but in the end it will asphyxiate you, blocking your energy and clouding your potential in the world. I have seen how ugly, hate filled emotions can harm the energy fields of yourself and others. A better way is to reel your ego back in, compassionately sort through your lingering hurts then set an intention to forgive. Not for anyone else, but for yourself.

Unfortunately for many people it is easier to hold onto complaints, revenge and bitterness than it is to surrender and forgive. But such attitudes poison your spirit and trouble your mind. *What we resist, persists.* Grudges cause blockages in your energy, they are emotional burdens. By contrast, when you forgive you release your negative energy which raises your vibration and literally lightens your load. Although forgiving will not change the pain of the past, it will have a profound effect on the way you think and feel *now*. It opens your heart to compassion and involves you transcending your sense of self inviting in a more expanded view of life and living.

Forgiveness is not only restricted to healing your wounds you can make it an integral part of your daily life. *Forgive and be the first to say you are sorry.* Just let go in the present moment. When you find yourself in conflict with another, decide not to worry about who is right and who is wrong, about whose game it was, even what it was all about. Take great pride in being the first to say sorry. Be so sure of yourself that you know you won't lose anything if you are the first to back down and apologize. You won't feel threatened, challenged or weak. You will feel accomplished, you will have showed how much you care. What it's about is irrelevant, you can apologize for arguing. You are showing yourself to be respectful, caring, mature, sensible and good. Just do it and see how it makes you feel - I trust when you've done it once, you'll want to do it again.

What it comes down to is the clarity of your heart, to stop defining yourself by those who have hurt you. Freedom lies within forgiveness - it is yours for the taking.

- *Calm your mind and center yourself. Begin to breathe deeply.*
- *Bring to mind events from the past that are linked to your forgiveness issues. What is your most hurtful memory? Allow any emotions to move through you*
- *Is this part of a pattern in your life? If so what might you be doing to perpetuate this pattern?*
- *As you exhale, imagine yourself letting go of any grudges. How will you feel if you are successful in your forgiving? How will you feel if not? Which would you prefer?*
- *Breathe deeply and simply let your deeper self tend to these things for you*

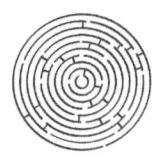

Day 54
Surprise

We could make our lives so much more interesting,
and develop so many new capacities,
if we sought to work with the unknowns of emergence,
rather than try and plan the surprise out of our lives.
- M.J. Wheatley

In every moment the Universe is whispering to you, bringing you messages and opportunities to step into the fullness of yourself. There is wisdom for you in the signs which surround you in every waking moment, personal messages just waiting to surprise you in each unfolding minute. Signs are all around you in your every day life, but are you listening? Whether you are conscious of it or not you are always encircled by signs; powerful indicators that encompass you bringing you a deeper understanding of yourself along with insights about your direction in life. They also reflect what is going on in your subconscious mind, what lies just beneath the surface of your conscious awareness. They can reflect your feelings and reveal your fears. However signs show up in your life they carry important messages about your present circumstances and your future whilst also acting as a reflection of where you are in your life right now.

We can never be prepared for everything. No one person can anticipate all of life, yet there are many people who try. They are holding on so tightly to the reins of their life that they plan the detail of every last moment, and live their lives oblivious to these signs. They know exactly what is going to happen, with whom and when, to the extent that there is no space left for anything to emerge. Their lives are so full in every waking moment as they busy themselves, planning, coordinating and controlling every last detail. *They plan the surprises right out of their lives.* When faced with obstacles undeterred they push through with a wellspring of determined effort. They fail to see that there might be another way presenting itself which would require less effort for similar results. *They fail to see their signs.*

Signs are always around you. There is never a time in your life when you aren't surrounded by them. The key is to slowing down or looking up enough from your daily plans to see them. Your signs come through the energy field of which you are an integral part. Everything around you has energy and that energy responds to your questions and your expectations. When you quieten your mind and really listen to subtle currents of energy swirling in the world around you, you can gain great wisdom. You allow your life to emerge, bringing with it surprises, the whispers of the Universe that give you understanding, insight and direction in your life.

- *Find some space to go deep within. Breathe slowly and deeply, allowing the outside world to fade away*
- *Ask for the courage to be open to your life, to allow signs to emerge*
- *As you exhale relax your resistance to the unexpected*
- *As you inhale make a passageway for everything that is larger than you to show you the way*
- *Begin your day*

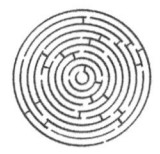

Day 55
The gift of choice

Every dawn, each man is offered, again,
the freedom of choice... while life remains,
there is always the opportunity
to remake the world.
- Jim Coleman

Each and every one of us has the gift of choice in our lives. We are free to make our own choices, even when we think we are not; there is always a choice. We can only consider things for so long before we become weighed down by all the information, the opinions and the options and it becomes harder and harder to make the choice. *The more we think we know the more we find out we know nothing.* We worry unnecessarily about our choices. There are no right or wrong choices, our judgement is merely an illusion. It doesn't matter which way we choose there is learning in all of our choices. So make no mistake everything you think or say or do is chosen consciously or unconsciously by you.

You choose where to be.

You choose how to act.

You choose what to say.

You choose what to do.

You choose who to be with.

You choose what to concentrate on.

You choose what to believe.

You choose how you show up.

You choose your energy.

You choose when to go along.

You choose when to resist.

You choose who to trust.

You choose who to avoid.

You choose to see.

You choose to ignore.

You choose to play small.

You choose to play big.

You choose what behaviors to emit in return to what stimuli.

You choose what to say to yourself about; self, others, risks, needs, rights.

You choose your thoughts.

You choose your choices.

You choose your life.

Above all, you choose you.

- *Center yourself and consider the choices that await you*
- *Enter into a deeper sense of knowing with yourself. Breathe into your core.*
- *Allow your intuition to bring you a sense of direction*
- *Breathe, get out of your own way and allow your knowing to surface. Choose*
- *Enter your day*

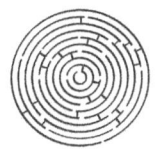

Day 56
Whole body listening

Let the rhythm and vibrations of the words
resonate through you. Listen with your whole body
and become attuned to the subtle energy fields.

Our energy issues are completely solvable, but we can't afford to remain deaf to the messages of our intuition. Intuition is directly linked to your core energy, your life force. It's job is to know every detail of what makes you tick, what makes your heart leap with joy and what drains your life-force until you are physically leaking energy from your very pores. *Intuition is a truth detector.* You can learn to tune into it. A good place to start is by whole body listening. I want you to start to listen now. Really listen. Listen to your inner voice of intuition. *I guarantee your energy will grow.*

Being able to sense and direct our life-force gets our positive energy moving; we exude it, attract it and can read it in others. It is our intuitive energy that drives our sense of well-being. We all give off energy whether we intend to or not, and our energy is either positive or negative - it is never neutral. Earlier in my consulting career one of my clients told me of his theory of people, he suggested that people fall into two types: there are radiators (those who radiate energy) and drains (those who drain energy). At the time, although a little simplistic, it struck a chord within me and energetically speaking, I now know his theory is completely true! This intuitive energy radiates from deep within the self, and reflects the quality of someone's being. Your energy reflects the quality of inner work you have done and ultimately the quality of relationship you have built with yourself. Have you managed to heal the anger within, the hatred, self-loathing we all feel from time to time and which can poison your energy, turning it toxic?

And what about those around you? Do you surround yourself with individuals who radiate positive energy or those who leave you feeling tired and drained?

The real power of whole body listening is that it gives us, at every moment, the ability to connect directly with our energy, allowing us to know when to radiate and when to protect our energy - giving us the ultimate capacity to influence our lives and ultimately to change our destiny.

- *Take a moment to close your eyes and go within yourself. Make a mental list of the people in your life, and imagine them sitting around you in a circle. Shift your focus from one person to the next, and connect with the energetic feeling that each one raises in you*
- *What's the first thing that comes to mind? How do you feel? Happy? Safe? Revitalized? Anxious? Afraid? Tired?*
- *Use your whole body to listen to what arises*
- *Spend a few minutes meditating on this and then open your eyes and write down the names of the people you've just been thinking about. Jot down the feelings that they inspire in you. Be brutally honest. (You can always write the feelings on a separate piece of paper for shredding afterwards if you are afraid someone may see it)*
- *Now sit back and notice what you have written*

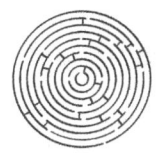

Day 57
Stepping into your power

It is never too late to be what we might have been.
- George Eliot

Think about your typical day. Do you have the same things for breakfast each morning? Do you buy a cup of coffee every morning on the way to work? Do you watch the same television programs, meet the same friends and have the same sorts of conversations? *When was the last time you made a conscious effort to do something different, to shake up your routine and invite a different energy into your life?*

Most of us are *slaves* to our habits and routines without even realizing it. As much as we like to think of ourselves as free agents embracing flexibility and spontaneity, we spend most of our time playing out the same repetitive patterns. We are creatures of habit which means that our behaviors and our energy can get stuck in familiar ways of being and it becomes alarmingly easy to allow mindless behavior to take over. This is true in our businesses as much as within our personal lives. Of course, our habitual activities play an important part in our daily lives. It is helpful for us to be able to complete complex tasks without really thinking about them e.g. when you first learned to drive, it took a lot of conscious effort for you to develop your driving skills, today you probably get into your car and drive without thinking; a highly efficient process, as it frees up your mental energy to be used elsewhere. If we had to spend time consciously engaging with our mundane activities we would have little time or energy left for anything else. *But when do we become conscious again?* We become so used to routine that we rarely stop to question what we are doing because it is what we are used to. We may believe it is the best way to do something, however as a result, *we limit our options.*

While there is comfort in familiarity, if we never stop to consider our choices, we risk living our lives in an automated fashion and trapping ourselves within a life which becomes boring and predictable. Usually as a result our energy suffers and we begin to tolerate discomfort in our physical, emotional and mental energy which then becomes our new "normal". Relying too much on our unconscious behaviors not only prevents us from seeing all the choices available to us, it also enables us to tolerate things which don't work for us, as we begin to accept them as part of our "normal" daily lives. *Time to step into the power of our energy.*

Tolerating anything usually highlights a place where your energy has become blocked, where you are not living your true potential. Energy blockages have *a real and negative impact* on your physical, emotional and mental health thus it is in your interest to become more aware of your energy and learn techniques to clear blocks moving yourself back into balance, alignment and flow.

The key to liberating your energy lies in living more consciously and mindfully. The first step is raising your level of awareness about what you are doing each day, to really notice what you do and also how that makes you feel. Once you begin to become aware of what you do, you naturally put yourself into a position of choice. You can simply decide if your behaviors are working for you or not. If not, then you can decide to change. Simple really. Changes don't have to be big to make a drastic alteration in your life, even small steps can have a meaningful impact and really shift your experience.

- *Spend today really noticing what you do - become more conscious in your actions and the choices you make*
- *Notice your energy. Allow it to bring you a stream of additional information*

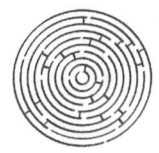

Day 58
Unconditional love

Love is, above all the gift of oneself.

The goal of our lives is not to master the rigid rules of perfection. The goal is to become impeccably aware of all our thoughts, feelings and actions so that we can achieve unity and harmony with everything we experience in life. We do this through unconditional love. It is through cultivating our love that we can embrace all the feelings and thoughts, the good and the bad, the light as well as the shade. We can then *integrate and become whole.*

There is much discussion about unconditional love and often I wonder if the true meaning has become mistaken. Unconditional love is not about a passive acceptance of whatever happens in the name of love. It is NOT a test of endurance, of tolerating unacceptable people or events in the name of love. It is about the deep vow to never, under any circumstances, stop bringing the flawed truth of our own reality into our relationships and our lives. It is about accepting ourselves and showing up in our energy as whole. allowing our energy to be seen. It is about being real and authentic. It is about daring to be seen.

The murmurings of your heart can inspire you to explore silent truths and find the willingness to bring more love into your life. It is as we move through the process of confronting our own shadow-like behaviors, that we evolve in our understanding of the wholeness within human consciousness. We begin to know love at a deeper level. We cultivate our compassion and realize that love is bigger than our individual selves. When we are in judgement of ourselves and others, negative feelings, critical thoughts and abusive behavior drain our life force. When energy is not leaked through negativity, boundless inspiration is available to us. We feel more connected and alive. Our heart energy expands as we move through our human notion of love to a more spiritual, deeper love that pervades our environments and can be found in unexpected places. It extends beyond our judgements, beyond our sense of self and embraces the very notion of life itself. *It is our part not merely to know this in our mental energy but to live this at a cellular level.* As Mahatma Gandhi stated "*We have to be the change we want to see in the world*".

In many ways we have no choice in the matter, as despite what we might think *we are all pulled towards what we feel is real*. It is as magnetic as the force of life itself. Being who we are releases an extraordinary power that without intent or design, affects the people who come into contact with it. When we can experience life in all its vitality we invite others to do the same and help them to be completely themselves. Once we accept ourselves with unconditional love we radiate into the universe expressing our light and warmth in all directions. Love transforms life and our love grows richer as we make the inevitable transition from conditional to unconditional love.

- *Sit quietly and let your heart open*
- *Allow the stream of your love to carry itself forward, filling your body with a glowing heart energy*
- *After a time allow your feelings to surface about love. Give voice to them. Acknowledge and accept them*
- *As you breathe in, breathe in love. As you breathe out, breathe out love.*
- *Notice what it would mean to allow yourself to be real*
- *Know that as you go through your day love is all around and within you*

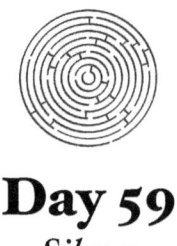

Day 59
Silence

Learn to get in touch with the silence within yourself
and know that everything in this life
has a purpose.
- Elizabeth Kubler-Ross

Although you may not want to live in a cave it can be helpful to shut the door on the noise of the outside world while you take some time to nurture your inner self. It is exceedingly difficult, if not impossible to get to know yourself without finding the space that silence brings into your life. You can't gain a firm footing with yourself if your interactions within are always filled with noise. It is silence that gives you the space for a new way of your being to emerge.

It is a phenomenon of our modern lives that for many people silence is almost unendurable. It makes us nervous. As adults we can become anxious that silence equals emptiness, and that in conversation it may be interpreted as low self-esteem or questionable intelligence. Many others feel silence signals a lack of participation, telling others we are not interested. *We fear people will think we have nothing to say.* We develop our careers with a belief that it's not okay to just sit there, you've got to say *something*. In social circles silence is an unwelcome guest, however *real interactions demand silence*. The more emotionally loaded the subject the more silence is required. This is true of our interactions with others as well as those we have with ourselves.

In conversations with ourselves as in life, less is more. It can be a good idea to breathe. Stillness is good. Walking can also help to keep your energy moving building momentum and distraction for your thinking mind. *You need to find the space between your thoughts* as this is the place where your insights can make themselves known. If you are like me, you may need to find your "off" switch. I often find there is no space between my thoughts, they come racing through my head putting my mental energy into a spin. They go so fast I can barely keep up, until I sit in front of water. I'm not sure what it is about the water but something about its breathless beauty stills my mind so I can connect to the silence within. Find your water, whatever it is that interrupts the habitual pattern of your thoughts and enables you to pause in stillness.

Even the briefest moment of silence is a way of coming into the present moment and a way of moving on. We all instinctively and intuitively know what to do with silence (and no, I don't mean fill it with noise!) We know how to be in silence, always just as we are, but with awareness, doing nothing, observing and allowing the fullness of what is. Silence allows us to *be* instead of *do*. Let silence like a zen koan, be your riddle. Fill your entire being with silence so that your reality may be interrogated, learning may be provoked and your relationships may be enriched. Allow your silence to move you beyond the doing... for now at least.

- *Find some space and be still*
- *Allow the silence to penetrate your thoughts and shift into your being*
- *Relax and meditate with the silence*
- *Simply be*

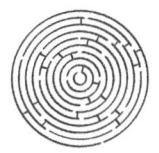

Day 60
Living life out loud

We are here to live out loud. Balzac

After the silence comes the noise. Our personal expression of life. In this busy world it is easy to lost track of what is important to us, to lose our connection with our energy and become consumed by the noise of everyone and everything else. We can forget the adventure of our own lives, that we are meant to harness the energy stream of our own lives and live our days filled with the vitality of our own voice. The *real magic* lies all around you, every moment of every day. It lies within your energetic expression that is just waiting for you to tap into it and work with it so you can live the life you were meant to live.

It is through your energy that you learn how to connect to your essential life force with *the power of your breath*. You can go deep within and find the truth that exists within your very core and live your life loudly from that place. You know that you are so much more than your five senses. You are a being of energy connected to all the energy in the Universe. You will notice when your energy is dense and heavy, making life difficult and exhausting for you and when life is light and flowing, when things are going well and life becomes easy. You can become aware of the energy of others and how it affects you. You will come to realize that sounding your way in the world, to express authentically who you are, must always come first.

As you tap into your own unique energy you will become a stronger part of the universal flow. Once you are in flow what you need flows easily to you. And as your body flows, you become physically healthier and stronger. You find your voice and express your energy with a clear resonance that sends a healing vibration out into the world. You become aligned in your energy, clear and resonant so that you naturally become louder in the world, without you having to do *anything*.

Become magnetic to others. Life becomes a fantastic adventure filled with possibilities, positive energy and amazing experiences. *You resonate wherever you go.* Best of all, all the positive energy you radiate out into the world is returned back to you threefold giving you a fabulous wave of energy from which to live your life. You are in flow with your energy and as you become more resonant in your energy, you naturally live your life from truth and joy. You are living life in alignment with your creative expression and living your life out loud!

- *Go for a walk into nature if you can and listen to the sounds of the birds, the bees and the animals*
- *Listen to the birds singing within the trees. Note how there seems to be nothing between their impulse to sing and their singing. Their sweet sounds resonate out clearly and uninterrupted into the environment*
- *As you breathe notice what you are feeling about living your life out loud - what hesitation keeps you from doing this?*
- *Meditate on releasing that hesitation*
- *Find your voice and as you breathe make a sound, however softly. Release the energy of your voice*

Recorded by the author, '**An Energetic Journey**'
is a free Guided Meditation that accompanies this book.

For your copy, go to: **https://rebrand.ly/AEA-Meditation**

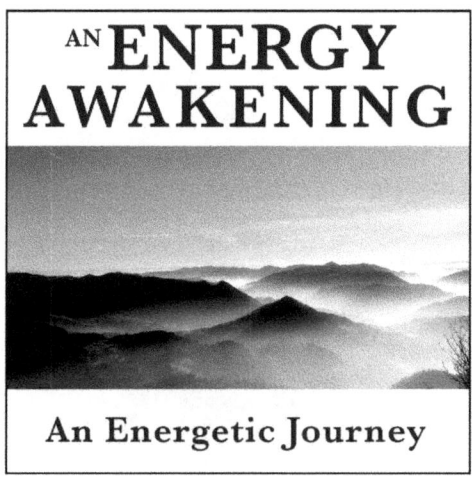

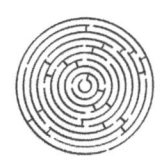

Part Four: Beyond the ego

Meditate. Live purely. Be quiet. Do your work with mastery. Like the moon come out from behind the clouds and shine!

- Buddha

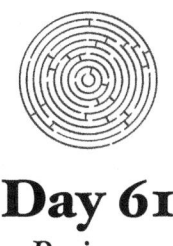

Day 61
Patience

It is better to be patient than it is to become one.

My mother was right, patience is not one of my virtues. I don't know about you, but my life seems to want to go faster as the years pass by. If I am not in the doing of something I wonder what it is I *should* be doing with my time. This is not always conscious for me and no matter how far I venture into my being, there remains a part of me who keeps trying to do more, faster. It is like I am trying to sprint to the finish line, and I get so excited about what is coming next that I miss the magic of this very moment. I become impatient to move on. I like my pace fast and become frustrated when things become slow. I want to scream inside when they appear to have stopped. *But why?* I have been on my learning journey now long enough to have learned differently.

When you find yourself in a place of waiting it can be a very difficult place to live. Fear wants us to act too soon. But patience, hard as it is, helps us to tune into our own rhythm and connect to the rhythms of others. I found this out whilst waiting to heal. I was not an easy patient. My general practitioner who was helping me to come down off immense doses of opiate medication gave me a six month plan to reduce my medication. I managed it within six weeks. The side effects were crippling yet somehow I felt liberated knowing I was fighting the pain. Had I waited, it would have been much easier. I am not sure where I thought I was going, or how I thought it would all be over within six weeks, it wasn't. Far from it. My body still needed time *to heal, to recover and renew.* I had merely plunged myself into an unnecessary physical crisis. As time moved on I learned from my mistakes. I learned that it was my fear and mistrust of my body forcing me into an unnatural rhythm with myself. I saw my body as an enemy that needed to be overcome, yet I learned that given enough time, I could surrender to a different reality. It is with the passing of time that we cease to remain in conflict, that most of our enemies cease to be enemies, because waiting allows us to reconnect to our humanity and see ourselves in them. Patience reconnects us to the truth within.

If you are feeling an urgency or impatience to move on, wait... and things that you fear will more often than not, shrink into a different energy enabling you to connect with *what is* in reality, of which you have no choice but to play your part. Most importantly, be patient with yourself. You make your life harder when you make impossible demands that you should do or be more than you can in this moment. Also you will help others around you feel better when you let go of your impatience with them. Let focused presence in the now take its place. You can almost always spare one single minute.

- *Sit quietly and meditate on the pace at which you like to live your life*
- *What does patience mean to you?*
- *How does waiting affect you?*
- *What lesson is there for you to learn in waiting?*
- *In the past what good things have arisen out of your waiting?*

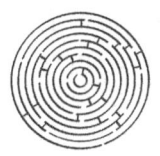

Day 62
Friends

One does not make friends, one recognizes them.

We all need people in our lives who share our dreams, help us conquer our fears, make us laugh and provide a safe space in which we can explore and grow. We needs friends who hold the threads of our shared history, and who in times of doubt can remind us of our best, most authentic self. I have been blessed in my life to have benefited from some deep friendships, they have been my anchor when the seas of my life became turbulent.

As friends we can each become increasingly powerful agents of one another's reality. *Friendship requests that we all keep our hands symbolically open;* so that you can give what you have and be open to receive what you need. It is this perpetual dance of friendship which creates long lasting and sustainable relationships. It is about sharing your love and your self with another. At the end of your days you want to leave this Earth knowing that you touched other people and allowed yourself to have deep and meaningful relationships. You want to know that you made a contribution and left the world a better place for you having been it. If you only managed to affect one person's life positively, then you have somewhere you know that you mattered.

Unfortunately it can be very easy to neglect this area of your life. You can so easily allow friendships to fall into the bottom of your to do list that you overlook the very people on whom you most depend. As a result your life can become stressful and lack the depth and richness that only meaningful friendships can provide. Create yourself a network of support, it is time and energy extremely well spent.

Nurture and care for your friends. Invest your energy with them to ensure that you radiate positive energy offering them a helping hand whenever they need it.

Develop a deep sense of connection where you are comfortable seeing and being seen; relationships where you can trust that you can reveal your innermost selves to each other. It is these deep relationships which re-ignite our energy. True friends offer us a port in the storm, a safe place to land when everything else around us is falling apart. They stand by us when everyone else has turned away. As a true friend yourself, ensure that you give as much as you receive and you will know the joy that arises in sharing your gifts and your life with others.

- *Sit quietly and ask yourself the following questions:*
- *Who is in my inner circle of friends?*
- *What kind of friend am I to them?*
- *What kind of support do I receive from them?*
- *What can I do to provide support to them?*
- *When was the last time I made time to connect with the people I find valuable?*
- *What can I do to inject some positive energy into these relationships?*
- *How can I appreciate them more?*

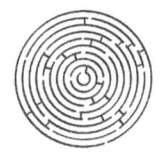

Day 63
Mindfulness

In any given moment, we are either practicing mindfulness
or de facto, we are practicing mindlessness.
- Jon Kabbat-Zinn

It is in our nature as a species to want to learn and grow and heal, moving towards greater wisdom and greater compassion for ourselves and others. Many would say that despite this, it is the challenge of our time to actually put these things into action.

Our life is a series of moments and our individual challenge is to make the most of the moments that we have. Generally speaking our moments are easily filled with stuff, intentionally and unintentionally yet it is *in the space that the magic really begins to happen.* It is within the space that we can begin to see that in the unfolding of our lives, all we have is moments. In reality we actually have nothing but a series of moments in which to live our lives. It is in the space that we begin a journey towards realizing who we really are and living our lives as if they really mattered. *And our lives do matter - perhaps more than we think.*

Mindfulness and conscious living is about developing our capacity for paying attention since it is this alone which refines our sense of awareness. It is this feature which distinguishes our potential for transformation and learning, both individually and collectively. We have the choice to grow, change and learn in direct relation to how we perceive ourselves to be. Jung distinguished our collective learning as the collective unconscious; a psychic system which we all inherit giving us access to a pre-existing reservoir of knowledge and energy.

Science has now caught up with Jung's ideas and has proven that energy exists as a field of interconnecting vibrations, a living matrix of energetic information of which we are all intimately connected. Your personal vibrations connect to this field sending ripples out into the Universe. You are always connected as there is no way to disconnect. *You are the energy, a living, breathing part of the field.* thus mindfulness and conscious living affects not only your own individual vibration but the vibrations of the entire planet - and no-one yet knows the outcome of raising our frequencies as a collective - but somehow it feels like a positive thing to do. The benefits are tangible individually, thus as a planet the effect must be amplified.

Regardless, as individuals we need to be present, to be awake to the here and now to ensure that we minimize our inherent risk of dying without actually fully living, without waking up to our lives and the amazing gifts of our intuitive energy.

- *Center yourself and enter into the moment you are in right now*
- *Breathe steadily and feel yourself become present with yourself*
- *If you find yourself wandering to somewhere else; to tomorrow, the future or the past, without judgement bring yourself back to the now*
- *Consider how present you are in your daily life - how can you be more present?*
- *As you enter your day, live your life in a mindful way*

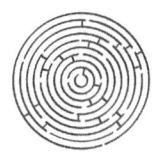

Day 64
No resistance

How you deal with your energy flow
has a major impact on your life.
When you resist, the energy has no place to go.

There really is no reason for tension or problems. Stress only happens when you resist life's events. If you are not pushing away or pulling towards you then you are not creating any resistance, you are simply present with your life. If you choose to live this way you will see that your life can be lived in a state of peace. When we take a step back from our lives it can be amazing to see what we end up doing with our will. There are many times when we actually assert our will into direct opposition with the flow of our lives. *If something happens we don't like, we resist it.* However when we inquire into our resistance at a deeper level we realize we are not resisting the actual situation but the experience of the event entering our energy field. We don't want the energy of the event passing through us and affecting us on the inside. We know it is going to have an affect on our emotional and mental energy so we try to stop it from passing through our hearts and minds.

Amazingly we can do this. The energy of an event transfers energy into our psyche, creating energetic ripples, much like when you drop a pebble into a pond. If you assert your willpower you can actually stop the energy transfer and that's what creates the tension and the blockage in your energy flow. You can drain your energy struggling with the experience of a single event, as we all know only too well. Eventually you will see that resistance is merely a tremendous waste of energy. Wherever you block your energy you close down. Over time the energies can build up to the point that a person's energy system becomes so blocked that they either blow up or burn out completely. If however, you don't let this energy build up inside of you, and allow each moment to pass through you unhindered, then you can be as fresh in every moment as if you were spending your days on vacation.

There are no problems. It's all about no problems, no stress, no tension and no burnout. The key is to relax and release. *Don't resist the energies as they pass through you.* Remain porous. If you have difficulty working with this, don't worry, just keep going. The path of least resistance is the path less travelled. It is the work of a lifetime to become that open to your life, that complete and that whole in your energy field.

- *Sit quietly and bring to mind a time when you completely resisted something that happened to you*
- *Notice what you did to resist and how this affected your energy*
- *What was the positive intention behind your resistance?*
- *Breathe deeply and allow yourself to feel compassion for yourself*
- *Inhale your compassion. Exhale your resilience into flow*
- *Inhale your compassion. Exhale your resilience into flow*
- *Allow*

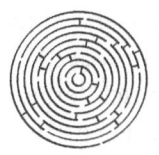

Day 65
Your vision

Your vision will become clear only when
you can look into your heart.
Who looks outside dreams;
who looks inside, awakens.
- Carl Jung

It takes vision to lead a life rich with meaning and purpose. It takes vision, both personal and collective to change the many dysfunctional aspects of our world which keep us unconscious, trapped and disengaged. Your vision is an essential part of the healing process. It is through this energy that you are able to imagine your future, to steer your psychic energy of consciousness and your actions towards a new vision. It is through these actions that you are able to consciously liberate yourself from the grip of the past and design a new future which makes all the difference. Your vision originates from the inside and it must be compelling to give you the energy to move into action and make it a reality on the outside.

A strong inner vision contains the light which leads us out of the darkness of internal confusion and distortion, into the clarity and thoughtfulness of an energetic world. It is here that we evaluate the conditions of our lives, recording our experiences, activating our inspiration and lighting our path and our purpose. The same energy stimulates our concern for all human beings, our sensitivity to injustice, ignorance or indifference and anything which prevents people from living in dignity, safety and security. It is through defining our vision that we are opened to the transcendent realms beyond ordinary awareness the subtle energies lying just beneath the surface of our lives. This expansion shifts our perspective and elevates our understanding to much broader levels bringing *profound insights*, allowing us to experience a much larger system of being than we have ever encountered. It is our inner or third eye which encourages us to begin to embrace the more abstract world of symbols, archetypes, dreams, fantasy and images. Just as one bit of a hologram clarifies the whole picture, each new thing we look at becomes immediately incorporated into our sense of wholeness, bringing more clarity to our internal picture.

From here, we encounter a panoramic view. *We can see beyond the horizon, beyond what our outer eyes can see.* We have entered a new dimension where we can see farther than before. Our vision becomes complete.

- *Step back from your life for a moment - in what areas do you have the most difficulty seeing the bigger picture?*
- *Describe yourself as you see you today. Describe how others see you*
- *Envision your ideal self*
- *How far are you from being the "you" you want to be?*
- *Allow the feelings, the worries and concerns to pass through you, breathe*
- *Breathe slowly and feel into the essence of you, of your infinite potential of you becoming all that you can be. It is certain*

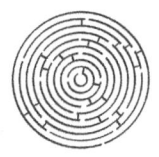

Day 66
Gratitude

Our inner soul is like a garden.
Gratitude is the healthy soil from which
the tree of paradise will grow,
and the birds of heaven will come to roost.
- Rose Crescent Sufis

Gratitude is one of the most powerful ways to express our caring and compassion for one another and to acknowledge the blessings of our lives. It is basically a nice place from which to live our lives. *Meeting the world with gratitude usually feels better than meeting it with resentment.* Some people live quite naturally with this understanding, while others take the steep path toward finding it. Like many of our emotions, both gratitude and resentment seem to perpetuate themselves. Every emotion has an underlying energy and it this energy which attracts a similar response in others. When you feel grateful, your good feelings tend to evoke friendly words from others and when you feel resentful and you express this, others can close up to you leaving you alone in your alienation.

Social psychologists and mind body researchers tell us that those who experience, express and embody gratitude more frequently than others tend to be happier, healthier, more forgiving, more helpful and less stressed. In other words *gratitude is not only good for your energy it is also good for your health.* When you are able to express and embody gratitude your body's chemistry actually changes, increasing the production of dopamine and serotonin, the so called *"feel good"* and *"happiness hormones"*. So you are not only sharing positive energy with others you are experiencing joy within yourself too.

Sometimes being grateful isn't always easy. If you find yourself without a job or someone you love dearly leaves you then it can be hard to see the positive, let alone give thanks. However, you can always be grateful for your inner strength and resilience that carries you through the tough times. When you find yourself in emotional uncertainty as we all do from time to time, sometimes a deeper appreciation of what you may be taking for granted can prevent a decline into negativity. *Gratitude nurtures your soul.* If you are grateful to be who you are and have what you have then you are on your way to peace of mind.

In order to fully experience gratitude you must be open to the landscape of its language which includes receptivity, kindness, appreciation, vulnerability, joy and acknowledgement. Gratitude invites you to revel in the blessings of your life, to wake up each morning to the possibilities of a new dawn and remain open to the new opportunities that lie within.

- *Focus on your breath*
- *As you inhale, contemplate a grateful thought*
- *As you exhale, breathe out a judgmental or stressful thought*
- *Breathe in positive energy, breathe our negative energy*
- *Count your blessings as you go through your day and you will notice everything that you feel thankful for*

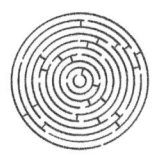

Day 67
Your creative DNA

Every child is an artist.
The problem is how to remain an artist once he grows up.
- Pablo Picasso

Creativity is not just for artists, it is for everyone. It is for business executives looking for a new strategy; it is for engineers trying to solve a problem; it is for parents who want their children to see the world in a new way and *it is for you*; for you to uncover the depths of your creative genius that hides somewhere within your soul.

Many of us wish we were more creative. We sense that we can become more creative, but are somehow unable to tap into our stream of creativity. Our lives can easily feel flat and predictable. Often we find that we have great ideas, or inspiring dreams for ourselves, but we are unable to bring them into being in actual reality. We may have creative longings to play a certain instrument, sing, dance or paint or we might yearn for a more creative way of life where we indulge an expanded sense of creativity in our professional and personal lives.

A return to our creativity is a spiritual journey. It is a reconnection with our expanded sense of self, a stark reminder of the dreams of our childhood and a return to an unrestricted flow of energy that rises up within us and returns to the world in a full, exciting creative expression. *Your creativity is instinctive.* You are already creative, you don't need to learn it as you would acquire a new skill. You merely have to remove whatever is blocking it, and get out of your own way. As you learn to recognize, nurture and protect your inner creativity you will be able to shift beyond the pain and creative constriction. You will learn ways to move through your emotions, recognize and resolve your fears and strengthen your confidence. You will find the spark within that connects to you a sense of expression which is far greater than anything you could think up by yourself. You will become the channel for creative endeavor opening your heart to a greater source of energy.

Your art is an act of your soul not your intellect. Living with creative passion can inspire you to find ways of being that open your mind and heart instead of ways that numb your sensitivities and keep you stuck in a rut. You can learn to be vulnerable, to make mistakes and to flow unencumbered into form. Some people are afraid of their creativity as they fear other people's criticism. Put your passion into expressing your creativity and don't worry about what others might say. Much of the value of your creativity lies in the energy, the sense of aliveness it brings you. Creativity sparks your enthusiasm for life and returns you to a world of possibility, a world where your true self can find its creative DNA and express itself without constraint. A world where you can bring the best of you out into all of creation.

- *Center yourself and contemplate any creative yearning which has not yet been fulfilled*
- *If you find yourself telling yourself that you are not creative - allow the thought to move through you and release*
- *Allow your creative self to step forward*
- *Breathe your way into your creative desire*
- *Give yourself permission to believe in your creative vision*
- *Live you life from your creative place today and notice the difference in your energy*

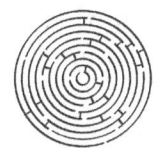

Day 68
The art of living

If I were to begin life again, I should want it just as it was;
only I would open my eyes a little more.
- Jules Renard

We all have something which pushes our positive buttons; something that takes us out of ourselves, something that gets us to forget our worries and challenges and make us smile from the inside out. It lies within the artistry of our lives. For me it is my children and sitting on the edge of my boat dock (I live on a lake). These are the things that can save my sanity on a really challenging day. They can reset my internal energy switch to happy and make me feel lifted in spirit and invigorated. But what is it for you? Over the years I have met many people with a startling variety of energizers from stamp collecting to sky-diving, from playing loud rock music to meditation. Whatever it is, make sure you have it, know it and use it whenever you need it. This is the stuff that makes you realize that *living is but an art*; everything you are worrying about isn't that important, whilst reminding you of the simple pleasures in life.

We all have a limited attention span, where we focus our energy is where we reap our rewards. We all know on some level that we should strive to get the most out of every day, to make the most of the time we have been given and not to miss anything along the way. We wonder what we need to do to be able to take in a little more; opening our eyes a little wider and listening a little more attentively? *To achieve mastery in the art of living is a lifelong preoccupation.* We are always learning. To see and be seen is something we all long for in our human connections. More importantly, we need to create space for our lives to be a container from which our energy can flow. We need to listen. There is a reason we were all born with two ears and one mouth! Listening is a key skill for most of us to develop, it helps to improve our relationships and it helps to improve our business skills. It is through listening to others you show them that you care, you care enough to give them your full and undivided attention. Listen to yourself, to everybody and everything. At this point, I don't just want you to be listening to the words either, I want you to be listening to the energy, to how people show up, to the things that lie behind the words which they may only be telling you implicitly. I want you to learn whole body listening where you can allow the words to resonate for you at a cellular level. You can begin to connect to the sacred energies of others, moving yourself into alignment with your environment and flow in your relationships.

Above all don't forget to listen to yourself. Create a sacred space. How you show up to your life, your relationship and your career counts and sets the tone for everyone else. It is in the listening that we grow. It is in the growing that we find our artist within.

- *Sit quietly and picture your life as a work of art*
- *Notice the sacred moments, the teachings, the love, the laughter and the joy*
- *Notice how you are showing up in your energy*
- *Breathe into your life today and allow what is sacred to find you*
- *Continue with your work of Art*

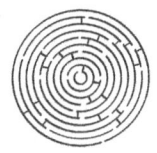

Day 69
Healing ourselves

I feel anything and everything my body wants me to know

I believe we can heal ourselves, I know this because I have done it myself. Long after I was written off by the medical profession and told I would never recover, I began very slowly to take the small steps to recovery. There were no guarantees it would work, in fact there were many times when my impatience got the better of me. I am not sure whether it was the power of my positive belief or my stubbornness not to live the rest of my life incapacitated which enabled my survival. I am more thankful than you may realize to say to you that today I have more health and vitality than ever.

I know at a cellular level that we are responsible for our own health. We are the stewards of an intelligence so powerful it can enable us to heal ourselves. The time has come for many more of us to know and experience this. *It is your right to heal.* It is your right to look inside yourself for answers. *Don't let anyone tell you differently.* No-one knows your body like you do.

Infinite quantities of energy are available to you. When your crown energy opens you receive direct healing energy, this not only heals your physical body but also radiates healing to others by its very presence. The truth is, spiritual healing comes naturally to all of us and it can be achieved every time we ground ourselves into our bodies, celebrate our vitality, claim our personal power, open our hearts, speak our truth, see the beauty in all things and have a desire to share this with all around us. In other words when we align our energy centers and open them to receive energy from the Universe, we can achieve spiritual healing in each of our energy centers.

You don't need to have any specific training to be a healing force within the world. The healing force is love, offered with the highest intention and the purest of energy from the crown. Chances are you have already experienced some healing energy; you will have done it as you held a child's hurt knee after they have fallen, or when you restored the confidence of others when they doubted themselves, or when you offered a kind word when no-one else knew what to say. This is all healing.

I'd like you to think of healing in the broadest terms. It may involve a complete resolution of pain or symptoms, a "cure" or it may not. On a profound intuitive level it also relates to the self-knowledge and growth achievable during illness or even as death approaches. Your body is most definitely your guide, it can tell you everything you need to know to heal. After working with many clients in their own healing journeys I have come to a profound realization; it is my belief that all physical illnesses can be cured and however painful it is to realize, I also know that not all people can.

Our crown energy center is more expansive than most of us realize. If we could only trust our magnificence, our crown energy would shine even brighter within our lives radiating out its divine healing potential.

- *Still yourself and see if there are any messages coming to you from your body*
- *Are there any areas of stress or strain which you need to attend to - physically? emotionally? mentally? or spiritually?*
- *If so, stop and face what is coming up for you*
- *Do what you need to tend to where you must go*
- *Breathe deeply and let your inner and outer attention go in the same direction*
- *Heal yourself*

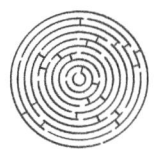

Day 70
Your personal vibrations

Don't get in the way of life with thoughts that don't move.
- Penney Pierce

From sunrise to sunset we are surrounded by waves, invisible frequencies that carry information in and around the world. About us, everything is oscillating. When it comes to your daily experience of energy, everyday reality presents you with another array of vibrations. In any ordinary day you move freely through energy which affects your physical body, your emotions and thoughts. It's normal for you to shift from the dense frequencies of the lower energy levels to the lighter frequencies of the higher energy levels. Many people I meet want to find a permanent way to remain in the positive energies and live their lives happier and more fulfilled. The most important thing for you to know is that *you can influence your personal vibration*, it is all possible.

From moment to moment your personal vibration naturally fluctuates as does the expression of energy which arises from the alignment of your different energetic levels. You are *a self-organizing system* and your personal vibration is affected by the vibrations of others. Your body is like a natural tuning fork, and when you come into contact with someone who is anxious and nervous, your energy will respond in empathy. Some people are more empathic than others, which means that they easily pick up the energies of those around them. Before they know it they can feel exhausted and drained. It can be like riding an emotional roller-coaster. Despite this, it is important to know that your personal vibration is generated from inside of you. Even empaths can transform their energy. Once you become more conscious in your energy you are less likely to be buffeted by the chaotic frequencies of energies existing within your environment.

By the time you reach adulthood, your natural vibration is often cluttered with the emotional and mental clutter you have picked up along the way. It is this clutter which can prevent you from resonating clearly and getting what you want in your life. You can choose to uncover it and radiate out more clearly anytime you want. So what are you waiting for?

Your energy state is a blend of contracted and expanded frequencies of your body, emotions and thoughts at any given moment. Your physical shape is an embodiment of these energies. *The more you allow your authentic self to shine through, the higher your personal vibration will be.* Although your personal vibration is affected by the energy around you, ultimately you are in control of your own energy and how you want to resonate out into the world is your choice. As you become more aware of your energy you can stabilize your home frequency, clear your blockages and open up to the flexibility and freedom inherent within your unique dynamic energy system.

- *Sit quietly and feel into the energy within your environment*
- *Contemplate the waves of energy swirling around and within you*
- *Notice how the energy affects you*
- *As you go through your day today, become more aware of your energy. Notice what happens to your energy in different environments and when around different people*
- *Observe your own personal vibration and how you are showing up to your world*

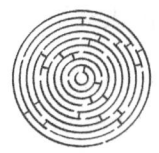

Day 71
Your inner leader

What you bring forth out of yourself from the inside out will save you. What you do not bring forth out of yourself
from the inside will destroy you
- Gospel of Thomas

Times have changed and leadership is undergoing an evolution. Leadership is no longer confined to those at the top of organizations, indeed it is no longer confined to those working within organizations. *Leadership is becoming an essential skill for us all;* it offers us many insights into how we as individuals become the leaders of our own lives, how we can harness the energy of our own internal leadership to enable us to show up with our whole selves to our lives, both professionally and personally.

Many motivational experts like to say that leaders are made, not born and yet in many ways I would argue the exact opposite. After working within corporate leadership development for many years I have come to realize that the skills of leadership are often about unlearning the things that don't work for you as a leader, rather than learning more of the latest tools and techniques. I believe we are all natural born leaders that have been deprogrammed somewhere along the way. As children we were natural leaders; we knew what we wanted from life and with a vivid imagination and a child's natural curiosity we were determined to get what we wanted. Think of the children you know, I bet they have clarity, the ability to inspire, motivate and influence those around them, to innocently engage others in helping them to achieve their goals. So why is it so difficult to do as adults? What happened to us along the way that means we need to read countless books, and attend leadership development courses to find our way forward?

I guess you could say we became socialized. As children we became used to hearing "No", "Don't" and "Can't". Our parents or other adults will have told us to be quiet, controlling our behavior until we learned what was acceptable to the adults around us. We went to school which reinforced this learning, and many of us will have gone onto further education, which reinforces compliant behavior, teaching us as students how to fit within an institutionalized system, succeeding by achieving good grades. Unfortunately our mainstream education system doesn't teach students how to become leaders; instead of learning to become creative, independent, self-reliant thinkers, most people learn how to obey and follow the rules, and as a consequence *we lose contact* with our inner selves.

The energy of your natural leadership lies hidden deep within, it remains there waiting to be rediscovered, however much your light may have faded over the years. Finding it requires a process of unlearning, the courage to explore your own inner attic, uncovering the dusty bookshelves where your childhood dreams lie and peeking inside to your very core. *It is time to honor your inner child,* to remember your unsocialized hopes for the future, of what mattered to you back then, what you wanted to achieve at the very heart of your soul. It is time to define your vision and your strategy for life and to lead your day from this place.

- *Take a moment to consider what has happened to your childhood dreams? To those "unrealistic" ambitions you embraced, the passion you had for becoming or achieving something great?*
- *Now is the time for them to rise again to the surface, to find their energy, to motivate you to make some different choices? Listen deeply*
- *Breathe and reconnect to your leader within, find ways to invite your inner leader back into your life today*

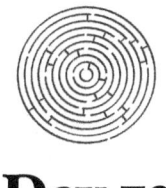

Day 72
Intuition

Intuition is our energetic diagnosis of an energy field
of information...
a sensing movement towards a future event.
- Carol Adrienne

Your intuition, already strong and insistent is prompting you to get ready for a new journey of discovery. A purpose deep within you is steadily unfolding, and it is not going to allow you to sleep your way through this lifetime. Prepare to be more awake in your life. Living using your intuition enables you a fast-track into your energy, that when mastered produces a thrill like no other. Intuition can make your life run smoother and be more fun, and I suspect it is going to be a critical skill of the future. Wherever I travel, I meet people whose physical and emotional lives are in turmoil. They can no longer rely on their careers, relationships or material possessions to bring them fulfillment in their lives - they sense that something profound and intense is happening within them, just underneath the surface, just out of reach. It is our intuition that can take us to the heart of what matters, it can cut through the noise providing calm in the face of chaos.

A number of myths surround intuition and one is that you need to be born with a "gift". Let's set the record straight now, *you don't!* I am living proof that you don't have to be born special or psychic to become a skilled intuitive, I developed my intuition much later in life. I have learned first-hand that developing intuition is a natural human ability and not the realm of a special few. We are all intuitive.

You are already intuitive, now, whether you respect, listen to or act on your intuition well, that's a different thing entirely!

Are you willing to know what might block the clear waters of your intuitive insight? Remember, the more honest you are with yourself the higher your level of accuracy will be. *Intuition is direct knowing.* It is incredibly effortless, the perception that connects us via our body to everything in the physical plane, through our heart and soul to all other souls and even extends to the core consciousness of trees, rocks, and mountains. Your intuition is immensely useful in the world for practical purposes; it keeps you safe, protects you from harm and teaches you to learn from your experiences but where it becomes priceless is as the vehicle for knowing, becoming and creating from your own unique and intuitive energy.

So many people embarking on this journey of intuitive development ask me what it is they need to learn, what techniques will help them to connect with their energy, when the truth is far simpler. Much of your intuitive development rests again with unlearning rather than learning. Of simply letting go of what is false, surrendering old habits that no longer serve us well, releasing the thoughts and ideas we cling to for security's sake. I have had many profound experiences on my journey to intuitive energy but more important has been the systematic letting go of what I know, of my attachments to who I think I am, of my ego and my sense of personal identity not to mention the things I *"should"* be, or do or have! *The more I clear the clutter from my field of personal energy, the more intuitive I become.* So far, it is still an ongoing process for me (yes, like most of us - there's a lifetime of clutter within), yet my transformation has been life-changing and yours will be too.

- *Listen to the messages from your intuition and notice how often is is right*
- *Learn to tell the difference between false messages and those you can rely on*
- *Commit today to build a relationship of trust with your intuition*

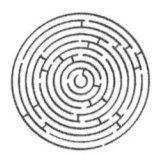

Day 73
Legacy

In the end, everyone is aware of this:
nobody keeps any of what he has,
and life is only a borrowing of bones.
- Pablo Neruda

Are you playing safe with your life? If so, why? *Haven't you figured it out that you are not making it out of life alive?* We are all going to die and once we know that at a deeper level the only question left is - *Are you going to truly live?* Our mortality may prove to be the ultimate inspiration and motivation for us to move into action in following our dreams and achieving our destiny. It can prompt us to consider our life in the wider context as we choose how we will live on in the hearts and memories of others once we have reached our deadline (*yes, pun intended*). We do this by finding our purpose, the meaning in our life, what it is we choose to stand for in how we choose to love, live and contribute to those that matter most to us.

In many cultures most people believe that legacy is something that occurs only after you die. Nothing could be farther from the truth. Every single one of us leaves a legacy, whether we do this intentionally or not. Your very existence has an impact on the world - so how do you want to be remembered? Whilst it is true your legacy will remain behind after your death it can be better appreciated as a process that is *active* within your life, an organic, ever evolving thread which weaves itself through the tapestry of your life. As the days of your life unfold your legacy is constantly forming. Its resources include who you are today and who you are becoming. It has an energy all of its own, continuously flowing, calling you to be all that you can be, preparing you to be the message in your own world.

Your legacy starts with you. It is your message to the future. It compels you to heed your call and find your passion, to fulfill your potential and keep your creative fires burning so that you will be able to pass the flame onto others. It requests that you differentiate yourself from the crowd and build your life to be resonant with others. It demands that you go to the edge of your learning, the edge of your comfort and step off into the great unknown to find your purpose. Purpose is what makes us human. Nothing gives vitality and energy to our lives like a worthy purpose. Find your fulfillment in serving others. Give your energy, time, talents and treasures away. Radiate positive energy. Don't just do, be.

Before you pass on, *it is your responsibility* to define your legacy to the world around you. Define it for yourself and use this to leverage your energy and empower yourself to live your best life!

- *Find a quiet place and meditate on your legacy - if you were to die today what is the legacy you would leave behind?*
- *If you had a lifetime to pursue your legacy what would be your intention?*
- *Consider your legacy from different perspectives: physically, emotionally, mentally, spiritually, financially, relationally, intellectually, logically, creatively, powerfully*
- *What matters to you? What are the messages you want to radiate beyond your lifetime?*
- *Breathe in and allow your responses to sink into your body*
- *Breathe out and know you can begin your legacy today*
- *Go out into the world and live your legacy!*

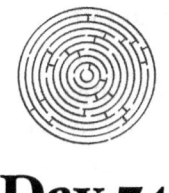

Day 74
Contribution

Life isn't about what you have,
it's about what you have to give.
- Anon

For you to be able to know what counts and what doesn't in your life, you need to know what meaning you are attaching to your life and ultimately what you are dedicating your life to. This is a very personal choice, no-one can tell you what is the right decision for you, you have to find it out for yourself. It is like an internal mission statement, something you hold in your heart and use as an internal compass to keep yourself on track. Disney's mission is "to make people happy" . Decide what it is you are dedicating your life to - it makes the rest much easier.

There is a great big wide world out there full of energy, life, vitality, experience, drive and excitement. See your community as part of your bigger picture. Getting involved means getting out there and becoming a part of your local community through contribution, co-operation, collaboration or just simply taking part.

We all know that if we throw a stone into a pond it creates ripples. We belong to a community and when we say something it causes ripples. Small or large our words and actions have an impact on those around us. Wherever we are in the world and whatever part we play personally or within our business, we need to realize that what we do has an impact. *It is no good pretending that we have no power to make a change;* we do. It is no good trusting others to make the decisions for us and hoping that they are going to be the right ones. We have to get involved and be a part of the process. We all have a part to play in the bigger picture. The more we do out in the world, the more we enrich our own experience and that of others. You will have developed many skills within your career, skills which can be put to good use in your community - so make some time to extend outwards - it will be good for you and it will be good for business life.

Make a positive difference in the world. Be generous with everything. Be generous with your generosity. You don't have to give money, your time and energy counts too. Find a place in your life to help others in some way. Whatever skills you have today, you will be able to lend them to others who need them. If you have the power to effect change for the better, use it. If you have influence, use it. You don't have to become a charity worker, you can make a difference in your own small way. It might take your imagination and creativity to work out how, but it is within your power to leave the world a better place for you having been in it. What are you waiting for?

- *Sit quietly and reflect on everything you are, everything you have become, all your gifts and skills that belong to you*
- *Imagine how you can use the fullness of you to make a difference in the world*
- *Consider your community - what is needed?*
- *In your inner vision, see yourself stepping out and giving back to your community. See with clarity how you can make a difference. Notice your contribution and the gratitude of those around you*
- *Sense into the emotions - how does it make you feel knowing you have many valuable gifts to share?*
- *What will it mean to you to contribute? Who will you become? How will it enrich your life?*
- *As the answers arise within allow yourself to feel into them and know intimately it is your time to step out and give something back*
- *Today, take the first small step into action*

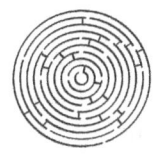

Day 75
Opening your eyes

*There was a time when I couldn't see the road ahead,
so I hit the accelerator, and the whole world opened up.
My dream is to expand my horizons.
It's much brighter out here than I expected.
- Lincoln cars advertisement 2007*

Awakening to a conscious life happens when we shift the way that we see and the manner in which we live our life. *Staying conscious is an ongoing process* that demands constant attention and commitment. I made a vow to myself a number of years ago to keep my eyes wide open and live a life of conscious choices, yet it is amazing how easily I slip into the dark well of being unconscious and need to consciously bring myself back into the light. It maybe easier for you, but I can guarantee it will take some effort. Consciousness can be challenging, as here you can't pretend you don't know - you see yourself and your life in the harsh light of day. There's no pretense, no illusion, just life as it is in all its glory, and there can be a lot going on.

As an extravert I believed I had a very open personality, I was happy to share just about anything with whoever I met and was not consciously hiding anything from view. However, opening my eyes and becoming more present with myself taught me that things were a little different. I realized there is so much is going on at any one time beneath what I show to the world, all my feelings, my thoughts, my hopes and expectations, so much complexity it can only be felt and experienced. When I articulate it into language it is somehow limited. My energy embraces many facets of my being, yin and yang, masculine and feminine including wisdom from previous generations,

I was literally full of things that cannot be said. It was not what I realized about myself that was startling more that I now understood this is something we all share as humans. *This is as true for you as it is for me.* Try it out and see. It changed the way I related to others. Now as I stand in the presence of another I am curious to go beneath the surface and I am able to stand before them long enough, with my eyes wide open, for their truth and wisdom to surface.

- *When someone is talking to you today, center yourself and drop within your body in the here and now*
- *Enjoy and experience deep silence within. Get in touch with your energy and bring some bright shiny energy into your eyes. Focus on the other person at all energetic levels. Focus on them as a soul full of wisdom, not just as a personality and give them your respect. Smile with every cell of your body*
- *Listen deeply to them. Let their ideas register deep within you, allow them to sink in effortlessly. Consider all their ideas openly*
- *Allow your own responses to arise gently from your very core*
- *Give them some space. Allow them to be. It is what it is*

Recorded by the author, **'An Energetic Journey'**
is a free Guided Meditation that accompanies this book.

For your copy, go to: **https://rebrand.ly/AEA-Meditation**

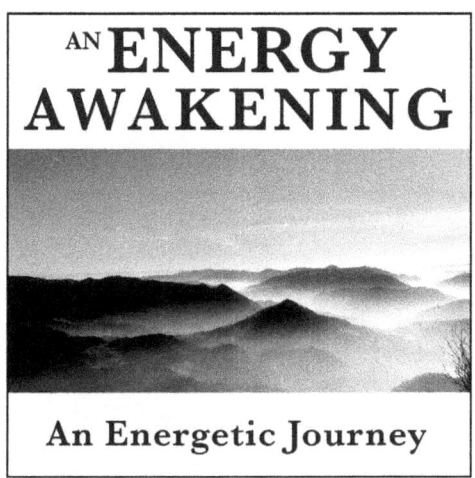

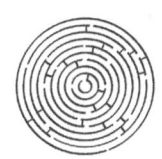

Part Five: Awakening

It is helpful to realize that this very body that we have, that's sitting right here, right now with it's aches and it's pleasures... is exactly what we need to be fully human, fully awake and fully alive.

- Pema Chodron

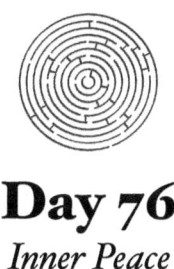

Day 76
Inner Peace

You can't find peace by avoiding life

We are not meant to struggle against life and ourselves. Every day we pass through situations that cause us stress, anxiety, worry and unhappiness. We often face problems, conflicts, demands and even emergencies at work, home or in our relationships. Our life can become an endless stream of drama and firefighting. All of these situations affect our energy, causing physical tension, emotional blockages and mental strain. It is in these situations that *a state of inner peace can be your life saver.* If you have a desire to make the world more peaceful, are you ready to take a good look and see if you can be more peaceful yourself?

Life happens, every day is full of unexpected circumstances, some good and some not so good. But they are all there for a reason and once you accept that fact, you can internally calm yourself and relieve your stress. If you allow yourself to *flow* with the circumstance, accepting it as necessary and important in your life, you can relieve the stress and become calm in the midst of the storm raging around you, no matter how strong and destructive it may seem. *It doesn't mean you like it;* it simply means you accept it and will work through it. In the end, the lessons you learned will make you stronger. In microcosm, peace is no further away than this very moment.

So what is inner peace? There is a lot of misunderstanding about what inner peace means. Some associate it with living a detached life in an ashram in India, not believing it is possible to have inner peace, and at the same time live an active life with work, family, daily chores and tasks. However, inner peace exists *independent* of external conditions and circumstances. It is a state that you cultivate within. *You can live a busy and active life, while your mind is peaceful.* In fact your energy *needs* you to find some space as an antidote to your frazzled life. If you find yourself in the midst of a chaotic existence it becomes essential for you to balance your life with some space for renewal, a time when you can soothe your soul and be open to the stillness within.

Imagine existing without a care in the world, without the feeling that there is something else you must take care of, manage or struggle against. *There is peace to be found within.* By letting yourself open up and discover who you really are you can give yourself the opportunity to live from this free space, from a place that honors you, that is whole and real for you without anything holding you back. This is how we are all meant to live; with freedom and clarity, a strong clear vibration of energy that resonates out into the world, free from blockages, conflicts and struggle. Open to the life that is unfolding around you. All of this is possible, it is a place that already exists within you, a spaciousness of awareness waiting for your embrace.

- *Sit quietly and drop inside of you*
- *Quieten your mind and find the space within*
- *Reconnect to the place of peace within*
- *Notice its qualities, the sensations, the feelings of your inner peace. Explore*
- *Contemplate how this peace is always with you, carried just beneath the surface, always open, readily available*
- *Languish in your inner peace. Embrace. Appreciate.*
- *As you enter into your day, take your inner peace with you as a companion*

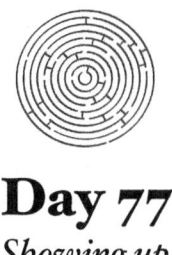

Day 77
Showing up

Bring yourself with you wherever you go and
show up with pure unadulterated joy

How are you showing up to your life? To your relationships? To your career? Are you bringing your self into your life? How you show up in your energy sets the tone for how you live your life. It determines the quality of your relationships and the quality of your experience on a daily basis. In short, it determines *the quality of your life.* Many of us never really consider how we are showing up, we suffer from a basic lack of awareness, and even when we begin to consider the questions above we can find we have not had sufficient practice in being ourselves to really know who "the self" truly is. If we spend our lives in self-doubt, moments in which we can find our true selves will be few. If much of our life is spent being afraid of the disapproval of others, or alone, we will also lose ourselves as fear and loneliness gain the upper hand. We can find ourselves meeting everyone else's needs and not our own. Time to return to the self and gain clarity to get ourselves back into our own lives.

Are you enjoying yourself? No-one else can tell you what to enjoy, you know at a deeper level, so your response can help you to reconnect with your essence. Joy is a high energy positive emotion and is now known to be a good indicator of health and longevity. You age slower and live longer. There are times in all our lives when we could do with lightening up a little, life doesn't have to be as serious as everyone makes out. We would all benefit from embracing a little more joy and laughter in our lives. It can help us to re-ignite our passion for life, bringing ourselves out to play in our daily lives. When you use the energy of joy you develop the capacity to enjoy fully what is before you. You learn to take delight in what you're doing, and not rushing through it and onto the next thing. *Cultivating enjoyment is a skill.* It requires you taking the time to refocus your energy and ask the question of yourself "What might I savor in this moment?". Doing this takes your thoughts away from an imaginary future and places them very firmly here in the present. You show up with positive infectious energy which demands that others come along for the ride. And quite honestly, it makes life a lot more fun!

Take this enjoyment challenge:

- *For the next day, resolve to taste and enjoy everything that you put into your mouth. Take the time to chew, enjoying the subtleties and intensities of aroma, texture and flavor, eating with presence and intention.*

- *Look around you, notice your surroundings. Look at the beauty of nature, the honesty of children and the joy of sharing time with friends and family. Consider the ground beneath your feet and the space above and around you. Take time to smell the roses. Notice the complexities within your own body, the amazing biology keeping you alive. Notice the detail. Be curious and amazed at how much passes you by each day - without you noticing.*

- *Before you buy anything at the supermarket, check out whether you will really enjoy eating it. Shop with the intention of creating joy for yourself and your family and cook from this place of joy too. Notice the difference.*

- *Do something, anything which brings you pure unadulterated joy. Do it simply for that reason and nothing else. Isn't it time you brought more joy into your life?*

- *At the end of each day, retrace your steps and remind yourself of everything you did which gave you joy. Be grateful for all the joy in your life today, Set the intention to find more joy tomorrow. You deserve it!*

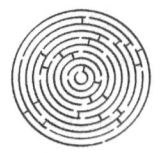

Day 78
Becoming whole

Evolution has become conscious of itself,
and what it wants is wholeness.
And that is an extraordinary place to find yourself.
- Ken Wilber

To enter into our lives fully, we must enter it with our full selves. We are all born whole and it is my hope that we will all die whole. However as we go through life our wholeness usually erodes. We are energetic human beings keeping balance in our different energy levels in a way we might consider to be our own unique orchestra. When all the instruments are in harmony there is symphony when even one element is off, we experience *dissonance*. Over the course of our lives, each of us takes a path that others haven't taken. We accept certain ways of doing because they fit us and we deny others because they were *just not us*. Over time, those paths and those choices make us into the person we are today. There are many limitations that we have come to live with that prevent us from entering into our lives more fully. For most of us we have become divided within; we like and accept some parts, others we push to the dark recesses within and pretend they are not part of our whole.

Most of us have also adopted roles that we play with others, often unknowingly. These roles become a version of reality that we identify with, and often these roles are not really us, they don't represent *the fullness of who we are. We are impersonating ourselves.* We are surrounded by expectations and standards concerning how we are supposed to act and what we are supposed to say. It is each of these expectations that limit our freedom to be in our essence who we really are and force us to show only parts of ourselves to the world.

Life presents us with problems that can't be solved with old answers. These are the problems that demand a change in our lives. There is nothing as frightening as facing the darkness within, our inner shadow. We will do almost anything to avoid having to look into the dark places of our soul. *There is no transformation that doesn't begin here in the darkness.* We merely have to find the gateway in and light a tiny candle in the dark, so that we can search for our future self, of who we are becoming and embody our wholeness from that place. It takes resourcefulness, patience and most of all, courage.

Becoming whole is a choice. It should be a choice that comes from your true self. Don't do this because you think it will make you more spiritual, do it because you know it is the right path for you. Being whole is about individual freedom and self-expression so you must *want* to be whole. Being completely who you are is not one thing but many. It is expressing yourself through conversations, behaviors and actions communicating to others how you *really* think and feel. It is about valuing your dreams and your inspirations. It is being willing to stand alone if your values differ from others. But more than anything else it includes the resonant energy of you, your own unique sense of rhythm. A willingness to breathe, think, speak, walk, laugh, cry and be silent at your own pace, in your own time and your own way. It is about being *you* in all places and at all times.

- *Center yourself and sense into the essence that is all of you*
- *Contemplate your whole self - are you ready to choose this way in the world?*
- *Are you ready to see and be seen?*
- *Notice any limitations which prevent you from showing up whole*
- *Release and let go*
- *Bring your parts together. Show up whole*

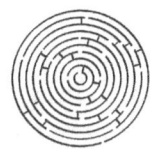

Day 79
Honesty and Integrity

It's not about what you do but who you are that matters

Being honest means that you speak your truth, by saying what is true for you. Not only do you *say* what is true but you must also *be* what is true for you. *You need to embody your truth.* True in the sense of being aligned with your energetic system physically, emotionally, mentally and spiritually. This brings your words into integrity with your energetic message, enabling you to be resonant and powerful in your communication. Honesty is not just a moral principle, when we avoid the truth we are cut off from ourselves.

Embodied honesty has an energy all of its own. It literally repels dishonest people away from you and attracts honest people to you. The same is true for the opposite; dishonesty repels honest people and attracts dishonest people into your life. So simply by becoming more radical in your honesty, the quality of the people you interact with will improve over time and in today's mistrustful society, other honest people will settle for nothing less. Don't fool yourself into thinking that nobody can tell when you are out of integrity either, we all know when someone is not being honest. It is easy to see when you are not congruent in your communication. Just watch the evening news, it's guaranteed that someone will put on a good show when faced with the media.

We all intuitively read each others energy, in fact we're rather good at it. So we all know when you are standing and walking with integrity, your actions match what you say you believe and value. You are literally *walking your talk.* Your values express what is important to you. Your family and friends will know you by your values, which are expressed not by what you *say*, but what you *do*. How you think and speak and where and with whom you spend your time. In our media society we are no longer easily fooled, after all *you can't relax and be yourself when you're hiding and pretending. It is way too stressful.* The reason a needle jumps around so much on a lie detector is that lying puts your energy under pressure, it is stressful. So is pretending, withholding, and misleading. If you are dishonest with a stranger, the event is only temporarily stressful for you, but in a close relationship, the deceit needs to be maintained, which causes you untold problems and prolonged stress. Become more honest in your very being and people will trust you more. You'll trust yourself, raising your confidence and self-esteem. When you're honest, you get to know *your real self* more. It takes a certain amount of discipline to be honest and in the demonstration of your honesty, you learn *you can count on yourself*. So another side-effect of being honest is that you will feel better about yourself. As my mother taught me many years ago, honesty *is* the best policy. Not because someone in authority says it is. Not because you might get found out. Not because it is the right thing to do. But because it balances your energy, brings you practical benefits and shifts you firmly into the flow of your life.

- *Contemplate your approach to honesty*
- *Consider your track record of integrity*
- *Allow any fears you may have about being radically honest to bubble up to the surface*
- *Exhale and release your fears*
- *If you were to be truly honest with yourself, what would that be like?*
- *If you were to be truly honest with others, what would that be like?*
- *Breathe and prepare yourself to be in honest throughout the day*

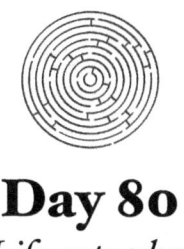

Day 80
Life as teacher

Your life is just one learning experience after another.

Learning and life are two coordinates which start and end together. Life is your teacher, it offers you an infinite array of opportunities to grow and learn and it brings you these experiential lessons one day, one challenge at a time. Your learning starts from the first day at birth and continues until you take your last breath. *Your whole life is an elaborate development program* which collects together a unique array of learning lessons to broaden your vision and take you into your own personal evolution. The learning opportunities unfold before you in a set of unique adventures bringing your learning to life and expanding your vision, calling you to be more tomorrow than you were today. It seems we all learn in two distinct ways; being who we are helps us to know more about this life and what we learn along our journey helps us to be more of who we are.

The *pace* at which we learn our lessons is up to us. Ultimately we have the freedom to choose to learn our lessons or not. Life has a way of compelling us forward, thrusting us into a variety of situations, all with the same theme, until exhausted, we surrender to the flow and we finally get it. We learn the lesson of the day. We are nourished in our learning by the very ground which appears beneath our feet, by the quiet teachers we encounter everywhere and by knowing that we have the *resilience* to overcome whatever life throws our way. Whatever doesn't break us makes us stronger.

We are responsible for the co-creation of our lives. We have sown our own seeds and nurtured even our most challenging lessons. So when something appears too challenging or overwhelming, it can help to remember the part we have played in bringing our lesson to life. Some of our lessons are exciting and filled with enthusiasm others are sheer heartache and can seem never ending. Each offers us something special, *a golden nugget of learning* which can enrich our experiences turning our life from the mundane to a masterpiece.

Learning it is not only an acquisition of knowledge. More than anything my life has taken me beyond the knowledge and deep into my own sense of knowing. My experiences whether resting in a hospital bed after the pain has eased or falling asleep with the words of my lover easing the worry from my brow, returns me to a simple naked truth that *the bareness of a moment can return us to ourselves.* My life has encouraged me to journey deep within my energy inviting me into the simplicity of a moment in which I understand that thinking, feeling, knowing and being are not only intimately connected but at their very core they (and me) are one.

- *Breathe evenly and deeply and detach from the outside world*
- *Contemplate your life as offering you a unique learning path*
- *How open are you to your learning?*
- *Lean into your life, embrace your learning*
- *Know at a deeper level that your life is your teacher and you are the student*
- *What are you going to learn today?*

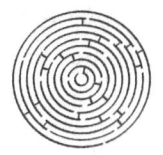

Day 81
Knowing why

He who has a why to live can bear almost any how.
- Friedrich Nietzche

Have you ever asked yourself *why*? Most people are born with an unconscious expectation that they are supposed to come into this world with everything already figured out, already put together and competent at living and loving. There comes a point in each of our lives when we have the unpleasant experience of realizing this is not the case, in fact we do and say things and we don't know why. We look at our lives and they do no resemble the pictures in our heads of how things should be turning out. This is not the life I ordered we cry. We wonder what we were thinking, or what lies behind our actions of why we do what we do. It can become a life-long fascination unpacking our selves to get to our why.

Firstly, *there is nothing wrong with you.* You've simply forgotten what you signed up for when you came here. Life isn't supposed to be easy, it isn't meant to be a smooth ride. It is designed to challenge you, so that you will grow into a more conscious, loving human being and all of this will get much easier when you uncover your why. So what is it that gets you out of bed in a morning? What makes your heart skip a beat and your heart grow lighter. Why are you doing what you are doing? What is it all for? Remember there is no single answer and whatever arises for you is neither right or wrong, *it is what it is.*

To experience enduring satisfaction we need to find some meaning in our life. For some, certainty comes easily, they have known from being very young that they wanted to be a doctor or lawyer; others can find it more of a challenge and wander through life searching for a real sense of meaning. Our *why* maybe a dream that beckons us forward in our lives. It maybe something that stays with us for a short time or an entire lifetime.

We grow into our why, one self at a time, questioning, declaring, aiming, missing and questioning again. The only way to know our why is to live through its many casings.

- *In Glastonbury England, the historic site of Avalon, a spiritual sanctuary since King Arthur's time, a lone hill overlooks the town. On it, an ancient tower called Glastonbury Tor stands alone as if guarding the small town, a sacred monument to the legends of the past, ushering in the energies of the future.*

- *In your mind's eye imagine that you have made the gentle climb to reach the Tor. As you look down on the town below, sense the potent energy surrounding you. Look out into the distance and as you do see your life spread its wings out before you. Scrutinize it carefully. Notice what feels most important - what is it that gives your life meaning now? What is your why?*

- *Next make your way back down the hill to a small wood, where a babbling brook makes it way through the trees. Sit down next to it. As you watch the water flowing, recall your most enduring sense of purpose, the why that represents the greatest value to yourself and others. Understand how you are investing your energy into this purpose. Know what it means in the larger, more expansive journey of your life.*

- *Breathe out into your own sense of sacred space and begin to embody your why…*

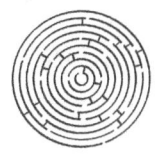

Day 82
Living on the edge

Love your edges, they point the way to your freedom.
All you have to do is to relax...
and lean into them.

As we move through the different levels of awakening we find that in the end our quest brings us, yet again, to the edge of our knowing. We can become masters at peeling away the different layers of our being until we come to rest in the center of our core. Living life as a learning journey takes us to our edges, where we are invited once again to step off into the unknown, having the faith to know that everything will unfold exactly as it is meant to, in its own time and space.

Every day we live naturally within the boundaries of our limits. It is our edges which teach us the limitations of our current way of life, they can also keep us from getting what we want or doing what we would like to do. Often this presents only a small problem but on rare occasions we can find ourselves facing a limit which gives us more of a challenge. It is not necessarily the limit itself which presents the problem but the very fact that we consider it to be a problem in the first place. *Some of our edges only exist because we think they do.* It is our perception of an edge, that brings us the issue and how we relate to it, how we experience it that can make all the difference.

Sometimes you are able to approach your edges with creativity. Other times you will be limited in very real ways that seem out of your control and present you with a rigidity you are forced to adhere to. Whatever edge you find yourself facing, there is a choice to be made. *You will be able to find the right solution when you step into the flow of your awareness.* When you lean into your edges and notice which represent your red light boundaries and which represent your opportunities for growth. It is through this practice of observation that you can also become clearer about those imaginary boundaries, those edges that you imagine to be real, yet on further exploration you find that it is merely your beliefs that give them power. Don't bring yourself unnecessary tension by finding more edges than are real.

Become aware of your energy. Practice sensing into the subtle energy field and allowing your intuition to push through into your awareness. *Listen with your whole body.* Cultivate every source of mental, emotional, spiritual and sensory information available, so that at each moment you can build a relationship with your edges. Don't allow your edges to be a source of tension in your life, merely allow them to ask you a question - it is after all your choice how you respond.

- *Find some space and come into the present moment*
- *Breathe steadily and notice what comes up for you as you contemplate your edges*
- *Visualize your next most compelling edge*
- *In your minds eye step out beyond the edge and explore what is there*
- *Inhale deeply and ask what part of your spirit requires attention*
- *Exhale deeply and though you may not have found your solution, give yourself the attention*
- *Relax, allowing your spirit to bring you your answers*

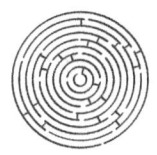

Day 83
Resonant energy

Change your energy, change your world.

All life is rhythmic; from the rise and fall of your breath to the beating of your heart. Your very life force can be seen as *a constant stream of pulsating energy*. Your body is a mass of vibrating, resonating energy that miraculously joins its frequencies to come together as a single ecosystem. It is your ability to function as a unified whole that depends upon *the coherence* of the resonance within you and it is your task to synchronize and enhance the quality of this resonance. It is this state of resonance within your bodymind which is a statement of your own unique health and vitality. It affects everything you think, say and do and it affects everyone around you.

Opening to resonance requires both grounding so you may establish a form of expression, coupled with an openness of breath which yields softness and flexibility. This is a delicate balance of letting and willing that allows you both to listen and respond at the same time. It is this resonance that has the potential to create an aura of wholeness within the etheric body, free from energy blockages or fragmentations. A clear energetic frequency that resonates powerfully into the energetic field.

A fragmented field makes fragmented connections, since when we interact with others our etheric fields become engaged. The most rewarding connections occur when there is resonance between vibrational fields. The greater our internal resonance, the more aligned our energy is and the more deeply we can connect to and resonate with those around us. So you can begin to see how changing your energy really does change your world!

The truth is that expression is the outlet for how we want our lives to be. *Life doesn't just happen to us* (although it can sometimes feel that way). The truth is that *we decide* how our lives are going to be - everything is up to us, we really are that powerful! It is our expression that facilitates this magic. This is such an easy statement to say that it can be hard to believe, yet when we realize that we truly are spiritual creators, our energy resonates at a higher frequency life really begins to fulfill our dreams.

Explore some different rhythms:

- *Listen to some music that makes you feel good. Dance*
- *Listen to some music that makes you relax. Sit quietly. Listen*
- *Listen to some music that reminds you of someone. Sing along*
- *Listen to a different genre of music from your normal music tasted. Expand your mind*
- *Listen to someone else's favorite song. Notice if it resonates for you*
- *Listen to your favorite song - and sing it out at the top of your voice (I find the shower a great environment for this!)*
- *Notice what types of music affect your moods and how. You can use this in the future to help lift your mood or adapt to a more positive state*
- *Find your own rhythm in the midst of your day. Resonate*

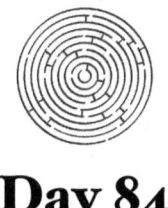

Day 84
Believing

Believing is all a child does for a living.
- Kurtis Lamkin

Henry Ford once said *"Whether you believe you can or you believe you can't, you're right!"* A very simple statement yet the implications are massive. Our beliefs are a very powerful force in our behavior, they have the power to create or destroy. It is our beliefs that determine how events are given meaning and they lie at the core of our motivation and culture. They are merely *decisions* we have made in the past about what is true or false about ourselves, other people and the way the world works. They provide the permission that supports or inhibits our capabilities and behaviors, yet for the most part we remain unaware of the beliefs that are affecting our lives.

Let's say that you have a belief that you are really ill. If that were true how much of your healing potential would you tap into? Not very much! Therefore the action you would take towards healing yourself would be rather half hearted, and the results you would get would be very disappointing. This reinforces what you thought in the first place, so the energy spirals around in a negative circle as a self fulfilling prophecy. What would happen if you held the belief that you could easily improve your health and bring yourself back to optimum health and fitness? You would tap into your full healing potential and the actions you take would be focused and positive. Therefore your results would be positive, giving you more evidence that you were in fact right in the first place. A spiral of positive energy, this time reinforcing a self fulfilling prophecy. How do I know? Well I lived it. The *turning point* in my healing came the day I believed I was no longer ill. It was the moment I knew that there was nothing standing between myself and my optimum health, everything changed. In reality nothing had shifted but my perception of events. My perception was everything. Changing your beliefs can be much simpler than you may think, however wanting to believe is not enough. For a belief to really serve you, it has to be something that rings true for you on every level, conscious and unconscious, down to the bone.

It's not only our personal life that is affected by our beliefs, it's all areas of our life. Our beliefs can shape, effect or determine everything from our intelligence, relationships, health, creativity even our degree of happiness and our business success. Your beliefs can empower or limit you. *So what are YOUR beliefs?* Finding out your own core beliefs can enable you to decide whether they are supporting you in your life or not. Shifting to an empowering belief can be as easy as finding out if anyone in the world has been able to achieve what it is you want to do - if they have, then you know it is possible. After all, if one person can do it, then anyone can... right?

- *Wherever you are sit quietly and contemplate your beliefs and how they shape your life*
- *Breathe. Relax. Be*
- *Notice your beliefs as you go about your day*
- *Find something that is limiting you and go in search of evidence to the contrary*
- *Change what supports you and let go of the rest*
- *When you can, go and talk with a child about how they see the world*

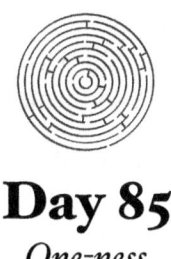

Day 85
One-ness

We are all connected in this dance of life

We are all interconnected. Despite our differences in nationality, ethnicity, age or socio-economic status, when we strip away our outer facades we are all essentially one. We all live within the wider energy field, a matrix that provides the container, as well as a bridge and a mirror for everything that happens between the world within us and the one outside our bodies. The fact that this field exists is changing everything we have believed as humans about our role in creation. When we look at life - our spiritual and material abundance, our relationships and businesses, our deepest fears and our greatest achievements we may be gazing squarely into the mirror of our truest, and sometimes unconscious beliefs. *Our life uniquely reflects who we are.* We are always intimately connected to the field, and to everyone in it. We don't have to do anything to connect, we already are an integral part of the field, already connected in this dance of life. Align yourself with the wider energy field. Everything that you could ever imagine and probably things you have never even considered are possible within this wider energy field. If your life is not all that you'd like it to be then you need to start the changes on the inside of you, within your own unique energy system. You need to become in your life and your business life the very things that you choose to experience in the world.

Cultivate your compassion. Compassion helps you to realize that everybody is one, they are each doing the best they can with the information and tools they currently have. Compassion alleviates blame and allows you to accept other people as they are despite their differences. The root of compassion begins at home with yourself. When you are compassionate and accepting of yourself you tend to be more accepting of others. It doesn't hurt to be nice and helpful

Make this your default setting in life, you may think it would take more energy to do this when in reality it will pay you back double what you put in. Always offering to lend a hand and being generally nice to everybody is really easy once you believe it is what we are supposed to be doing anyway. You may be helping others, you are also helping yourself since we are all connected as one.

Begin every day smiling and thinking the best of people, seeing where somebody might need a hand instead of hurrying past. It's about seeing life from someone else's perspective, being sympathetic if they have problems (remember you don't have to solve them!) It means making the effort to make sure people around you are okay.

- *Center yourself, turn your attention inwards and feel into the energy within you. The energy which lies deep within your physical body, enabling you to breathe, heal and grow.*
- *Sense the pulse of your life deep within*
- *Now turn your attention outside of your body. Become present in the moment and notice the energy around you. Hear the sounds of others, people, animals or birds. Listen to the sound of the ground beneath your feet. Sense into the color of the energy swirling around you. Feel the energy all around.*
- *Sense your contribution to the energy field. Step back and notice how we are all connected in this dance of life.*
- *Meditate on this one-ness.*

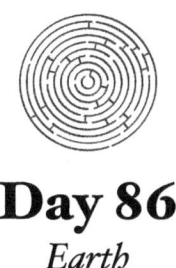

Day 86
Earth

A place we all call home... which means
you are home no matter where you are.

What you do and how you live matters more than you might think. What you choose to do in the next five minutes, and the energy with which you do it, contributes to the difference between the destruction of our world and the opportunity we have to return to Eden. *The future rests in your hands*, and the stakes are getting higher with each passing minute. It is time for us all *to wake up* to our consciousness, to become aware of our intuitive energy and our connections to the wider field. It is time to live our lives *passionately* and wide awake and to develop conscious relationships as radiators of positive energy.

It is time for us all to stop adding to the chaos, the destruction of our Earth and become an *active* part of the solution. This is not just about sympathizing and understanding our global problems but actually moving into positive, affirmative action. If you want your life to feel right, to be good, successful and mean something then you have to give something back. *You have to reinvest in life for future generations.* Why? Because it is too easy to watch from the sidelines, thinking it is someone else's problem and the reality is if we don't take some real decisive action, this extraordinary planet of ours which we all call home is doomed, taking us with it.

The truth is most of us have too many possessions, too much food, too many places to go, too many things to do in our business. All of which we tell ourselves is so important, when all we are really doing is making ourselves feel more important. In fact, many of us are exhausting ourselves in the pursuit of having it all. Come to terms with the reality that *you can have some of what you want, but you can't have everything*. Maybe what you have today is enough. What a radical thought.

The Earth is your home, so treat it well. Cherish and nurture the people in it, no matter who they are or where they come from. We are all part of the human race. *It is time that we all stood together and joined hands in celebration of our beautiful planet.* Don't wait for someone else to come and save us. We are at the edge right now. This is the evolution. These are the times. We are the people. You are critical.

- *Pause with all the doing and embrace your being in the present moment.*
- *Breathe deeply and allow yourself to be completely at home on this Earth. Consider the overwhelming beauty of our planet, the majestic mountains and the expansive oceans. All the many different and colorful forms of life. Your family, friends and everyone and everything that matters to you needs the earth to survive. Including you.*
- *Be with yourself. Be with your life. Just be.*
- *What do you notice?*

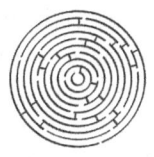

Day 87
Following the light

The light in me sees and knows the light in you.

There is a very touching story in the Talmud when a Rabbi asks his students "How do you know the first moment of dawn has arrived?" After a long silence one student responds with "When you can tell the difference between a sheep and a dog" The Rabbi shakes his head no. Another speaks up, "When you can tell the difference between a fig tree and an olive tree." Again the Rabbi says no. No-one else answers. The Rabbi breaks the silence and slowly begins to respond "You know the moment of dawn has arrived when you look into the eyes of another human being and see yourself".

We all have a light within us, and whilst you are unique and no-one is quite like you, or sharing your life path, *you are not alone.* Everyone is on the same journey. We all share the same fears, confusion and pain. We are not alone.

When you find the courage to *shine your light* others will respond. The more deeply you are able to go within, the more powerful and effective you will be when you come out shining brightly into the world. Just as bright lights are difficult to ignore, so are people who have found their source of their inner light. *It is your purpose in life to allow it to shine.* Once you do, you will find that others are attracted to you like bees around a honey-pot. Just as you will be attracted to the light that shines brightly from within another.

First you must reconnect to your light and enable it to glow deep within. Establish yourself in that state of inner stillness, feel a sense of calm wash over you and connect to that brilliant light which glows deep within your centre. The most important commitment you can make to yourself is to include some form of inner connection to your light as a regular part of your life.

Live your life from this place, allow your energy to shine out through you and into your environment. Your light is for sharing it is a source of positive energy for yourself and others. Go about your day glowing from your inner source, spreading radiance wherever you go.

- *Sit quietly and breathe you way into your center*
- *Simply breathe until you feel your heart open and the warmth of the bright light which radiates deep within*
- *Feel into your light, don't think about it just feel it - feel into the heat and the light. Notice how it glows, shining light on your dark places, bringing lightness deep within*
- *Navigate your day by taking your light along with you. Allow yourself to shine just a little more than normal*
- *Notice what happens to your energy*

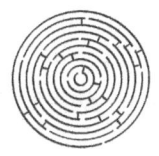

Day 88
A sense of purpose

The purpose of life is... a life of purpose.

You have a physical body and a life, but *are you alive with a sense of purpose?* No matter how much you may drift across the landscape of your life you are not an aimless soul. You and your life have a purpose, whether you are conscious of this or not. You are here on this planet for a reason. When you become clear about your life purpose a feeling of inner contentment begins to develop within you. You realize that *every* experience in your life has been preparing you for finding your true path, propelling you forward towards fulfilling your ultimate purpose in life.

At this moment you may be in a stage of your developing purpose, but no matter how blocked you feel - I want you to know that *you are on track.* Your purpose will have already made itself known to you through what motivates you, what interests you, what you resist and what frustrates you. It can be glimpsed in those qualities you admire in others. It can be seen in those abilities you have that you don't even think are special - those things you do so easily without even thinking about it. You are almost always working on your purpose when you lose track of time and shift effortlessly into flow with life.

You are a self-organizing system. Your purpose is to create life out of who you are and who you are becoming. We are all born to be directors of energy. It is through our energetic development that our purpose becomes clear. Once we can breakthrough the limitations of the lower energy levels and rise to the challenges of the higher energetic levels, life gets a whole load easier. We can follow our energy inwards into the heart of our true self, to learn more about what we need and want, what energizes us and what drains our energy. We can also use our energy to extend outwards into the resonant field, radiating and sharing an exchange of positive energy with everyone we meet.

Your purpose is not a thing, place, career or even talent. Your purpose is to be. Its essence lies in how you live your life, not what role you choose to live. Your purpose is to be found in each moment as you make the choices to be completely who you really are. *To grow in your energy is to become more purposeful.* You will be more aware of the consequences of your actions, and naturally move into alignment in relationship with other people and things. Learning more about your energy enables you to wake up to the essence of yourself and become more conscious of everyone and everything. You will find freedom in your energy as you begin to realize that there is a purpose for everything that happens in life and that ultimately, we are all connected in this dance that we call life.

- *Today watch for signs, coincidences and synchronicities*
- *Ask yourself the following question about every experience today "If this event had a message for me, what would it be?"*
- *At the end of the day reflect upon the experiences of your day. Spend some quite time meditating on the question "Why am I here?"*
- *Allow your life to show you a sense of purpose*

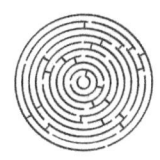

Day 89
Dare to dream

So many of our dreams seem impossible,
then improbable, then inevitable.
- Christopher Reeve.

Very often we define ourselves by what we dream of. As a child I dreamed of being rich and famous, of going down in history, of making a real difference with my life. Yet we can find that when our lives shape us differently and reality stares us in the face, we may think we have failed, that we are settling for less because we weren't good enough to become or have what it is we yearned for. We find our dreams only added to our sense of disappointment and somewhere along the way we forget to dream at all. *Our energy shrinks* and *we become smaller* than we need to be.

We are complex human beings in an even more complex world, there is so much we don't know and don't yet understand about the world of energy. It is an exciting field where there is so much more to be discovered - it is evolving continuously, as are YOU. *It is never too late to find a new dream or visit one that has been long forgotten.* Know that you will never understand everything there is to know yet, there is always more waiting for you on the horizon. Dare to dream of everything you can, *develop a passion for what's possible.* Once you begin to envision a bigger future for yourself, and you take the first step into action, the energy field will organize itself around you. The subtle energies will bring you a stream of information to guide you in your endeavors. Your energy will become charged with possibility, expanding your field and filling you with a vitality and re-energizing your life. Don't take my word for it - do it and notice the difference in your energy. I can tell you much about energy but until you experience it for yourself, you will not understand the sheer power available to you at any moment of the day. I want you to keep an open mind and find some time to begin to develop your awareness of the *subtle energies* which are around all of us all of the time.

Open yourself to the potential of your own unique energy blueprint and your connections to the field. Sense it in yourself, connect to it in others and read the energy of a situation, it can open up a whole new stream if information to support you in your life and your business. Use your dreams to charge your energy, expand into your life and follow your dreams wherever your energy may take you.

- *Envision for yourself the largest, most outrageous dream you can*
- *Watch yourself achieving it. Notice the difference it brings to your life. How alive it makes you feel.*
- *Sense into the energy around your dream - feel into it at a cellular level*
- *Now stretch your dream a little farther, make it a little bigger*
- *Come out from behind yourself and voice the impossible, enter into the realm of fairytales where you only expect the best*
- *Charge your dream with the energy of intention. Commit to follow wherever the pursuit of this dream will take you.*
- *Smile from the inside and allow your inner child to guide you into your dream...*

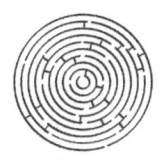

Day 90
A life worth living

Don't worry about what the world needs.
Ask what makes you come alive and do that.
Because what the world needs
are people who have come alive.
- Howard Thurman.

People who lead fulfilling lives have generally found a sense of home in what they do. They have a philosophy of life that connects them to a larger vision. They know themselves well and have developed a relationship with themselves based on trust, compassion and love. They show up *whole* to their lives and relationships continuously learning and finding themselves at a deeper sense of knowing with each passing challenge. They accept that life is a continuing challenge and they allow themselves to enter into *the rhythm and flow* of their own lives. *They know that their life is about more than them.* They are not driven by urgency, competition or the demands of the ego. They are happy to have found an internal harmony and are able to engage fully in their lives bringing their strengths and passions alongside their vulnerabilities and weaknesses.

You have your own place in the world. You have your own dreams and expectations. You have your own definition of what would make a life worth living for you. *Don't adopt anyone else's definition*, this is one time you have to get clarity of your own. The earth is working *with* you. You will be attracted to the energy of your own special place where you will find the silence that will heighten your senses. You don't need to seek it out. If you are willing, you will find yourself naturally guided to people, places and anything that helps you to connect to the Universal energies.

As you begin to feel into and awaken to *your energy* you will feel more alive, because energy is alive. You will become aware that you are a wonderful, magnificent, wise being who has the capacity to *change the world*. To use your life as a positive contribution and really make a difference. You will harness the powerful energy that is running through you and begin to utilize it to its full potential. Every time you radiate positive energy you affect others, who in turn will affect others. It creates a ripple effect that goes out into the energy field and touches everyone it meets.

The world is awakening and *you are the world*. It is time for us to stand in collaboration and community, to rejoice in being on the Earth together. It is time for us all to awaken our energy, to wake up to the energy of our lives and to live passionately and consciously. Don't wait for someone else to come and save us. We are all we've got. The future rests in your hands and the stakes are getting higher. Your planet needs you. What you do and how you live is more important than you might think. Your contribution matters. It depends on you to take the next step. Make no mistake, the time is now and you are the one.

- *Sit quietly with a trusted friend*
- *Breathe deeply and meditate on the awakening of the world and the awakening of you. Connect into your awakening and the raising of vibrations around the world. Let the wordless feelings stream through you*
- *Open your heart and open your mind to the energies of awakening*
- *After a time, speak to your friend from the heart. Share your journey of who you are and who your becoming.*
- *Allow them their turn. Be fully present. Allow their words to resonate deep within. Listen to them and be filled with their presence*
- *Be thankful for the blessings of your life*

BE RADICAL. BE REAL. BE RESONANT.

Recorded by the author, **'An Energetic Journey'** is a free Guided Meditation that accompanies this book.

For your copy, go to: **https://rebrand.ly/AEA-Meditation**

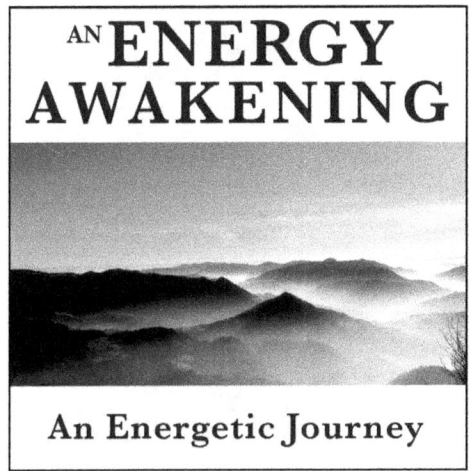

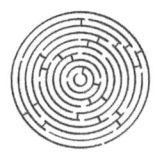

Epilogue

You've made it. Take a breath. Now take a deeper breath. This is not the end it is the beginning.

Imagine that you are 100 years old and preparing yourself to die. Before taking your last breath you are given a fantastic gift; to return to the person who is reading this page and share with them your wisdom, your advice to help support them in their quest to be a better person and to awaken to living a more fulfilling and worthwhile life. The older "you" understands with clarity what was really important in your life and what wasn't; looking back it is obvious where you have tended to lose your way or become distracted from your true purpose.

What advice would this "wise old you" have for the "you" today who is reading this page?

Find yourself some space to write your answers down. Allow the words to resonate through your entire body, feel into them and recognize them for the truth they contain.

Once you've written the words down the rest is simple. All you have to do now is to live it. Make it your commitment to yourself to embody this advice, to practice it at every opportunity until it becomes a habit.

You see you already know what is missing from your life. You already know what it would take to become fully engaged in your life, to open your eyes and your heart a little wider and live your life a little larger. Use that wisdom today. Don't wait until tomorrow as tomorrow never comes.

Don't look ahead, it is time to look behind; to look back from your old age at the life you would like to live. To define your legacy and begin to live it fully and freely today. In this moment. Right now.

You are here. You are awake. You are alive. The beauty is you have everything you need to succeed. Your energy is waiting. Don't let anyone or anything stand in your way. This is your life. Live it fully. It is time to allow the energetic river of your life to flow freely.

About the Author

Jayne Warrilow is the founder of JW International, a global coaching and development company with a focus on resonance as the key driver of individual and organizational success. She is one of the world's most exclusive business coaches, and her clients are by invitation and referral only.

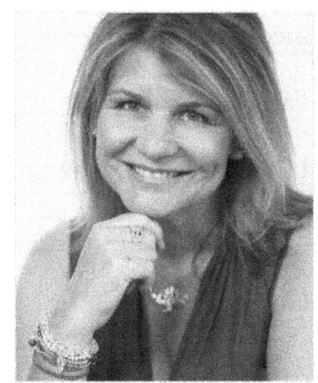

Jayne has worked with CEOs and Senior executive teams around the world, best selling authors, trailblazing coaches, entrepreneurs, thought leaders, millionaires, celebrities and people who simply want to make a difference.

An expert on business and leadership, Jayne specializes in helping coaches build conscious, seven figure businesses, to go beyond coaching and build a body of work that positions the coach as a trusted authority in their field. Her clients are passionate, powerful and prosperous with a track record of success, individuals looking to play even bigger. A natural edge-walker, she has enabled leaders worldwide to take a stand, create radical new rules of business, generate systemic change and transform their leadership for game-changing results. Her unique methods have brought the flow of innovation from the C-Suites of global corporations to the home offices of business owners igniting the charge that leads to high octane business growth.

Born and raised in England, she has worked with leading organizations and individuals in the United States, Europe, Asia,

Australia and Latin America. Jayne now lives and works out of the Greater Los Angeles Area, California.

Jayne would love to hear from you - so connect with her on social media or send an email to jayne@jaynewarrilow.com and say hello!

Facebook: https://www.facebook.com/JWIntl/

Linkedin: https://www.linkedin.com/in/jaynewarrilow/

Twitter: https://twitter.com/JayneWarrilow

Google+: https://plus.google.com/u/0/+JayneWarrilowJWI

www.ingramcontent.com/pod-product-compliance
Lightning Source LLC
Chambersburg PA
CBHW070655100426
42735CB00039B/2147